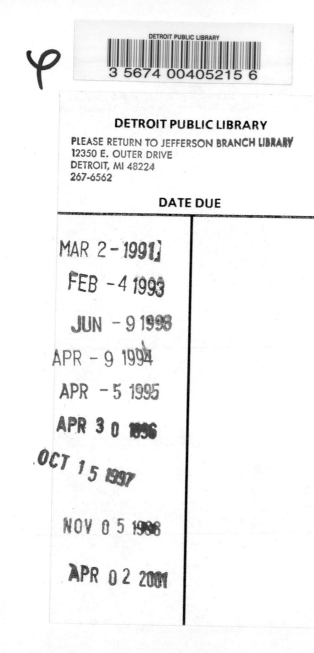

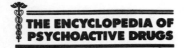

THE ENCYCLOPEDIA OF PSYCHOACTIVE DRUGS

IN 25 VOLUMES
Each title on a specific drug or drug-related problem

ALCOHOL	***Alcohol*** *And Alcoholism*
	Alcohol *Customs & Rituals*
	Alcohol *Teenage Drinking*
HALLUCINOGENS	***Flowering Plants*** *Magic in Bloom*
	LSD *Visions or Nightmares*
	Marijuana *Its Effects on Mind & Body*
	Mushrooms *Psychedelic Fungi*
	PCP *The Dangerous Angel*
NARCOTICS	***Heroin*** *The Street Narcotic*
	Methadone *Treatment for Addiction*
	Prescription Narcotics *The Addictive Painkillers*
NON-PRESCRIPTION DRUGS	***Over-the-Counter Drugs*** *Harmless or Hazardous?*
SEDATIVE HYPNOTICS	***Barbiturates*** *Sleeping Potion or Intoxicant*
	Inhalants *The Toxic Fumes*
	Quaaludes *The Quest for Oblivion*
	Valium *The Tranquil Trap*
STIMULANTS	***Amphetamines*** *Danger in the Fast Lane*
	Caffeine *The Most Popular Stimulant*
	Cocaine *A New Epidemic*
	Nicotine *An Old-Fashioned Addiction*
UNDERSTANDING DRUGS	***The Addictive Personality***
	Escape from Anxiety and Stress
	Getting Help *Treatments for Drug Abuse*
	Treating Mental Illness
	Teenage Depression and Drugs

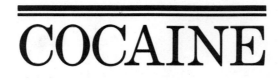

COCAINE

GENERAL EDITOR
Professor Solomon H. Snyder, M.D.
Distinguished Service Professor of
Neuroscience, Pharmacology, and Psychiatry at
The Johns Hopkins University School of Medicine

———————

ASSOCIATE EDITOR
Professor Barry L. Jacobs, Ph.D.
Program in Neuroscience, Department of Psychology, Princeton University

———————

SENIOR EDITORIAL CONSULTANT
Jerome H. Jaffe, M.D.
Director of The Addiction Research Center, National Institute on Drug Abuse

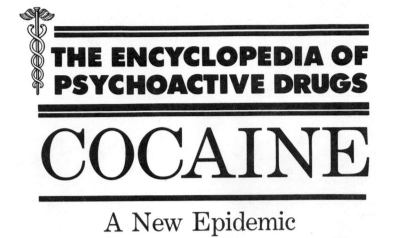

THE ENCYCLOPEDIA OF PSYCHOACTIVE DRUGS

COCAINE

A New Epidemic

CHRIS-ELLYN JOHANSON, Ph.D.

University of Chicago Medical School
Drug Abuse Research Center

1986
CHELSEA HOUSE PUBLISHERS
NEW YORK
NEW HAVEN   PHILADELPHIA

SENIOR EDITOR: William P. Hansen
ASSOCIATE EDITORS: John Haney, Richard S. Mandell
ASSISTANT EDITORS: Paula Edelson, Perry Scott King
CAPTIONS: Jeff Freiert
EDITORIAL COORDINATOR: Karyn Gullen Browne
ART DIRECTOR: Susan Lusk
ART COORDINATOR: Carol McDougall
LAYOUT: Noreen M. Lamb
ART ASSISTANT: Victoria Tomaselli
PICTURE RESEARCH: Ian Ensign

First printing

Library of Congress Cataloging in Publication Data
Johanson, Chris E.

  Cocaine, a new epidemic.
    (The Encyclopedia of psychoactive drugs)
    Bibliography: p.
    Includes index.
    Summary: Examines the history, dangers, and increasing appeal of cocaine
abuse in America.
    1. Cocaine habit. 2. Cocaine—Physiological effect. [1. Cocaine. 2. Drugs.
3. Drug abuse] I. Title. II Series.
RC568.C6J64   1986   362.2'93   85-25969
ISBN 0-87754-765-3

Chelsea House Publishers

Harold Steinberg, Chairman & Publisher
Susan Lusk, Vice President
A Division of Chelsea House Educational Communications, Inc.

133 Christopher Street, New York, NY 10014

345 Whitney Avenue, New Haven, CT 05510

5014 West Chester Pike, Edgemont, PA 19028

Photos courtesy of AP/Wide World, Art Resource, Bettmann Archives, Columbia
Pictures, 800-Cocaine Hotline, Fitz Hugh Ludlow Memorial Library, Gaia Books
Ltd., Michael Aldrich, Museum of Natural History, New York Medical Academy,
New York Public Library, Phoenix House, Timothy Plowman, Dr. R. E. Schultes,
UPI/Bettmann Newsphotos, Washington Post.

JUN   '87

CONTENTS

Foreword 9

Introduction 13

1 What Is Cocaine? 19

2 The Effects of Cocaine on the Body 29

3 Cocaine Use: History, Patterns, Trends 51

4 From the Field to the User 65

5 Scientific Studies of Cocaine's Effects 73

6 Treatment For Cocaine Abuse 81

Appendix: State Agencies 94

Further Reading 100

Glossary 101

Index 105

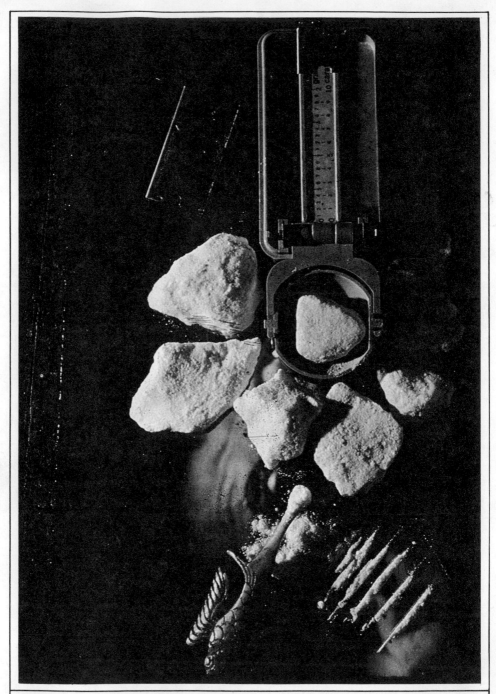

Bolivian rock cocaine being weighed and cut into "lines" for inhaling. The Bolivian coca crop, although illegal, is that country's most valuable export, bringing in almost $2 billion a year.

FOREWORD

In the Mainstream of American Life

The rapid growth of drug use and abuse is one of the most dramatic changes in the fabric of American society in the last 20 years. The United States has the highest level of psychoactive drug use of any industrialized society. It is 10 to 30 times greater than it was 20 years ago.

According to a recent Gallup poll, young people consider drugs the leading problem that they face. One of the legacies of the social upheaval of the 1960s is that psychoactive drugs have become part of the mainstream of American life. Schools, homes, and communities cannot be "drug proofed." There is a demand for drugs—and the supply is plentiful. Social norms have changed and drugs are not only available—they are everywhere.

Almost all drug use begins in the preteen and teenage years. These years are few in the total life cycle, but critical in the maturation process. During these years adolescents face the difficult tasks of discovering their identity, clarifying their sexual roles, asserting their independence, learning to cope with authority, and searching for goals that will give their lives meaning. During this intense period of growth, conflict is inevitable and the temptation to use drugs is great. Drugs are readily available, adolescents are curious and vulnerable, there is peer pressure to experiment, and there is the temptation to escape from conflicts.

No matter what their age or socioeconomic status, no group is immune to the allure and effects of psychoactive drugs. The U.S. Surgeon General's report, "Healthy People," indicates that 30% of all deaths in the United States

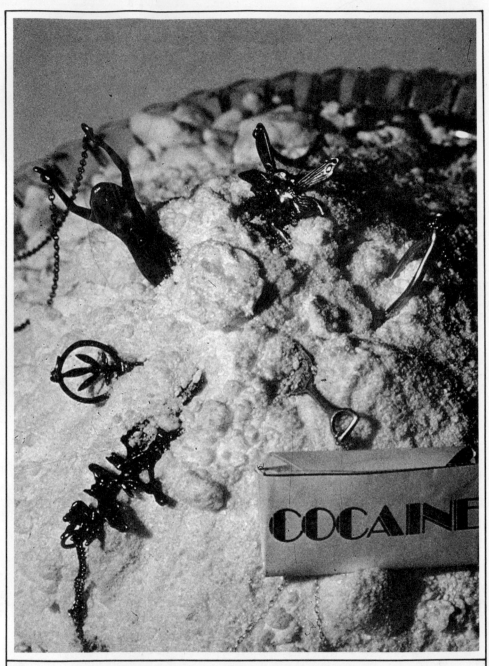

An estimated 5 million Americans use cocaine regularly and about
22 million have tried it at least once. Cocaine is one of the more expensive
illegal drugs of abuse. A kilogram of the drug (pictured above) costs between
$25,000 and $55,000, depending on its purity—most cocaine is diluted
with additives.

are premature because of alcohol and tobacco use. However, the most shocking development in this report is that mortality in the age group between 15 and 24 has increased since 1960 despite the fact that death rates for all other age groups have declined in the 20th century. Accidents, suicides, and homicides are the leading cause of death in young people 15 to 24 years of age. In many cases the deaths are directly related to drug use.

THE ENCYCLOPEDIA OF PSYCHOACTIVE DRUGS answers the questions that young people are likely to ask about drugs, as well as those they might not think to ask, but should. Topics include: what it means to be intoxicated; how drugs affect mood; why people take drugs; who takes them; when they take them; and how much they take. They will learn what happens to a drug when it enters the body. They will learn what it means to get "hooked" and how it happens. They will learn how drugs affect their driving, their schoolwork, and those around them—their peers, their family, their friends, and their employers. They will learn what the signs are that indicate that a friend or a family member may have a drug problem and to identify four stages leading from drug use to drug abuse. Myths about drugs are dispelled.

National surveys indicate that students are eager for information about drugs and that they respond to it. Students not only need information about drugs—they want information. How they get it often proves crucial. Providing young people with accurate knowledge about drugs is one of the most critical aspects.

THE ENCYCLOPEDIA OF PSYCHOACTIVE DRUGS synthesizes the wealth of new information in this field and demystifies this complex and important subject. Each volume in the series is written by an expert in the field. Handsomely illustrated, this multi-volume series is geared for teenage readers. Young people will read these books, share them, talk about them, and make more informed decisions because of them.

Miriam Cohen, Ph.D.
Contributing Editor

11

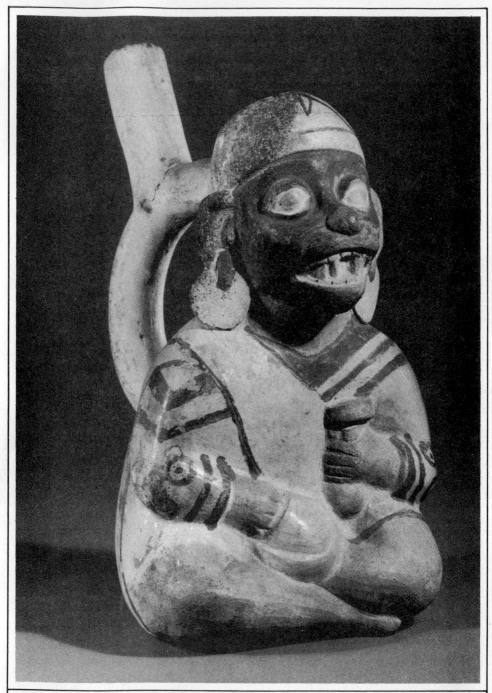

A 1500-year-old ceramic figurine depicts a Peruvian deity holding a bag of coca leaves. The ancient Indians of Peru believed coca was a gift from the gods and used the plant in religious ceremonies.

INTRODUCTION

The Gift of Wizardry
Use and Abuse

JACK H. MENDELSON, M.D.
NANCY K. MELLO, PH.D.
Alcohol and Drug Abuse Research Center
Harvard Medical School—McLean Hospital

Dorothy to the Wizard:

"I think you are a very bad man," said Dorothy.
"Oh, no, my dear; I'm really a very good man; but I'm a very bad Wizard."
—from THE WIZARD OF OZ

Man is endowed with the gift of wizardry, a talent for discovery and invention. The discovery and invention of substances that change the way we feel and behave are among man's special accomplishments, and like so many other products of our wizardry, these substances have the capacity to harm as well as to help. The substance itself is neutral, an intricate molecular structure. Yet, "too much" can be sickening, even deadly. It is man who decides how each substance is used, and it is man's beliefs and perceptions that give this neutral substance the attributes to heal or destroy.

Consider alcohol—available to all and yet regarded with intense ambivalence from biblical times to the present day. The use of alcoholic beverages dates back to our earliest ancestors. Alcohol use and misuse became associated with the worship of gods and demons. One of the most powerful Greek gods was Dionysus, lord of fruitfulness and god of wine. The Romans adopted Dionysus but changed his name to Bacchus. Festivals and holidays associated with Bacchus celebrated the harvest and the origins of life. Time has blurred the images of the Bacchanalian festival, but the theme of drunkenness as a major part of celebration has survived the pagan gods and remains a familiar part of modern society. The term "Bacchanalian festival" conveys a more appealing image than "drunken orgy" or "pot

13

party," but whatever the label, some of the celebrants will inevitably start up the "high" escalator to the next plateau. Once there, the de-escalation is difficult for many.

According to reliable estimates, one out of every ten Americans develops a serious alcohol-related problem sometime in his or her lifetime. In addition, automobile accidents caused by drunken drivers claim the lives of tens of thousands every year. Many of the victims are gifted young people, just starting out in adult life. Hospital emergency rooms abound with patients seeking help for alcohol-related injuries.

Who is to blame? Can we blame the many manufacturers who produce such an amazing variety of alcoholic beverages? Should we blame the educators who fail to explain the perils of intoxication, or so exaggerate the dangers of drinking that no one could possibly believe them? Are friends to blame—those peers who urge others to "drink more and faster," or the macho types who stress the importance of being able to "hold your liquor"? Casting blame, however, is hardly constructive, and pointing the finger is a fruitless way to deal with problems. Alcoholism and drug abuse have few culprits but many victims. Accountability begins with each of us, every time we choose to use or to misuse an intoxicating substance.

It is ironic that some of man's earliest medicines, derived from natural plant products, are used today to poison and to intoxicate. Relief from pain and suffering is one of society's many continuing goals. Over 3,000 years ago, the Therapeutic Papyrus of Thebes, one of our earliest written records, gave instructions for the use of opium in the treatment of pain. Opium, in the form of its major derivative, morphine, remains one of the most powerful drugs we have for pain relief. But opium, morphine, and similar compounds, such as heroin, have also been used by many to induce changes in mood and feeling. Another example of man's misuse of a natural substance is the coca leaf, which for centuries was used by the Indians of Peru to reduce fatigue and hunger. Its modern derivative, cocaine, has important medical use as a local anesthetic. Unfortunately, its increasing abuse in the 1980s has reached epidemic proportions.

The purpose of this series is to provide information about the nature and behavioral effects of alcohol and drugs, and the probable consequences of both their moderate use and abuse. The authors believe that up-to-date, objective information about alcohol and drugs will help readers make better decisions as to whether to use them or not. The information presented here (and in other books in this series) is based on many clinical and laboratory studies and observations by people from diverse walks of life.

Over the centuries, novelists, poets, and dramatists have provided us with many insights into the beneficial and problematic aspects of alcohol and drug use. Physicians, lawyers, biologists, psychologists, and social scientists have contributed to a better understanding of the causes and consequences of using these substances. The authors in this series have attempted to gather and condense all the latest information about drug use and abuse. They have also described the sometimes wide gaps in our knowledge and have suggested some new ways to answer many difficult questions.

One such question, for example, is how do alcohol and drug problems get started? And what is the best way to treat them when they do? Not too many years ago, alcoholics and drug abusers were regarded as evil, immoral, or both. It is now recognized that these persons suffer from very complicated diseases involving deep psychological and social problems. To understand how the disease begins and progresses, it is necessary to understand the nature of the substance, the behavior of the afflicted person, and the characteristics of the society or culture in which he lives.

The diagram below shows the interaction of these three factors. The arrows indicate that the substance not only affects the user personally, but the society as well. Society influences attitudes towards the substance, which in turn affect its availability. The substance's impact upon the society may support or discourage the use and abuse of that substance.

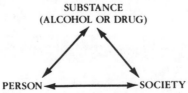

SUBSTANCE
(ALCOHOL OR DRUG)

PERSON ← → SOCIETY

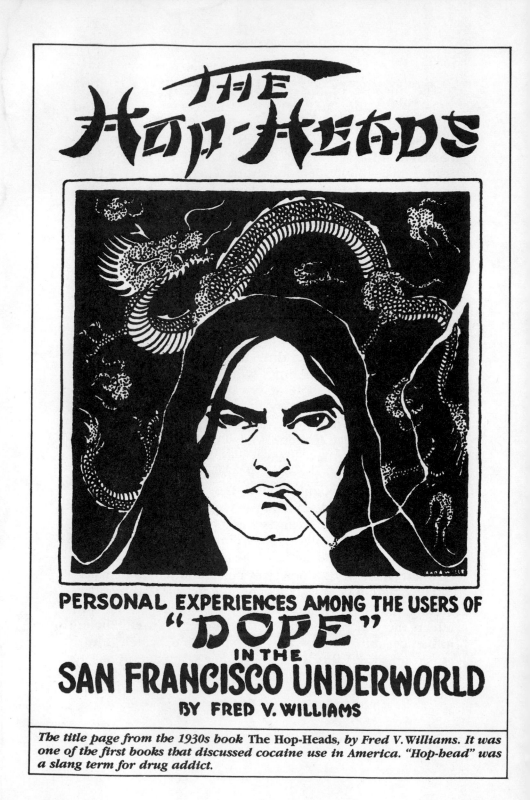

The title page from the 1930s book The Hop-Heads, by Fred V. Williams. It was one of the first books that discussed cocaine use in America. "Hop-head" was a slang term for drug addict.

Although many of the social environments we live in are very similar, some of the most subtle differences can strongly influence our thinking and behavior. Where we live, go to school and work, whom we discuss things with—all influence our opinions about drug use and misuse. Yet we also share certain commonly accepted beliefs that outweigh any differences in our attitudes. The authors in this series have tried to identify and discuss the central, most crucial issues concerning drug use and misuse.

Regrettably, man's wizardry in developing new substances in medical therapeutics has not always been paralleled by intelligent usage. Although we do know a great deal about the effects of alcohol and drugs, we have yet to learn how to impart that knowledge, especially to young adults.

Does it matter? What harm does it do to smoke a little pot or have a few beers? What is it like to be intoxicated? How long does it last? Will it make me feel really fine? Will it make me sick? What are the risks? These are but a few of the questions answered in this series, which, hopefully, will enable the reader to make wise decisions concerning the crucial issue of drugs.

Information sensibly acted upon can go a long way towards helping everyone develop his or her best self. As one keen and sensitive observer, Dr. Lewis Thomas, has said,

> "There is nothing at all absurd about the human condition. We matter. It seems to me a good guess, hazarded by a good many people who have thought about it, that we may be engaged in the formation of something like a mind for the life of this planet. If this is so, we are still at the most primitive stage, still fumbling with language and thinking, but infinitely capacitated for the future. Looked at this way, it is remarkable that we've come as far as we have in so short a period, really no time at all as geologists measure time. We are the newest, the youngest, and the brightest thing around."

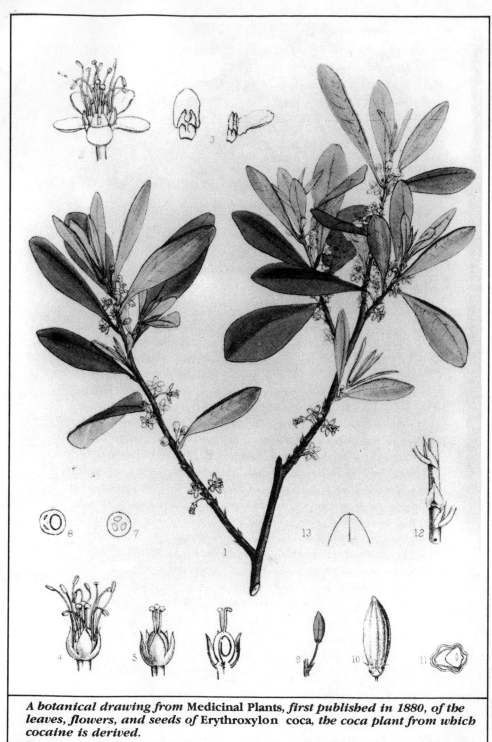

A botanical drawing from Medicinal Plants, *first published in 1880, of the leaves, flowers, and seeds of* Erythroxylon coca, *the coca plant from which cocaine is derived.*

CHAPTER 1

WHAT IS COCAINE?

*T*here are few drugs of abuse that have received as much public attention as cocaine. In recent years lead articles in news magazines, national television shows, and major documentaries by such well-known people as the oceanographer Jacques Cousteau have focused on this controversial drug. But cocaine is by no means a new drug. Cocaine has been used in the New World since before the Spanish Conquest. In fact, there is archeological evidence that the Indians of the Andes mountains in Peru have been using cocaine-containing substances for over 3000 years. The type of cocaine used today has been available since the 1850s, and its addictive properties were appreciated in the 19th century.

The lore about cocaine and its effects is widespread and colorful, and yet, other than the work of Austrian psychoanalyst Sigmund Freud in the 1880s, its effects and pharmacological properties were not systematically studied until the 1970s. Though today much more is known about cocaine, many misconceptions still prevail, such as the one that claims that this drug is relatively harmless. This book will provide readers with accurate information about how cocaine works and what effects it has on the body. It will also discuss the seriousness of cocaine abuse and describe the possible treatment for those people abusing it.

Cocaine is a white crystalline alkaloid powder derived from the coca plant, *Erythroxylon coca*, that grows in abundance in the Andes mountains of South America. (An alkaloid is a chemical that contains nitrogen, carbon, oxygen, and hydrogen and is found in plants.) The drug is extracted from the plant in two simple steps. First, the leaves along with sulfuric acid, kerosene, or gasoline are placed in a press and crushed to form a mash, or paste, containing up to 90% cocaine sulfate. Second, to remove any remaining impurities, this paste is treated with the solvent hydrochloric acid, which produces the white, crystalline cocaine hydrochloride.

Cocaine hydrochloride can be introduced into the body by sniffing, swallowing, or injecting to produce its characteristic effects. Only pure cocaine can be smoked, however, and thus the hydrochloride portion of the compound must be removed, or freed, by a process known as freebasing. This is done by first mixing cocaine hydrochloride with sodium bicarbonate (baking soda) or water and ammonium hydroxide. The cocaine, which is referred to as a base, is then sep-

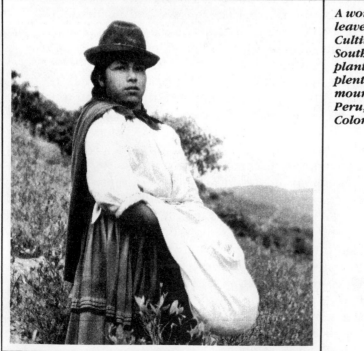

A woman picking coca leaves in Bolivia. Cultivated primarily in South America, coca plants are especially plentiful in the mountain valleys of Peru, Bolivia, and Colombia.

arated, or freed, from the water by using a fast-drying solvent such as ether. Unlike cocaine hydrochloride, the cocaine base is not water soluble and can be ingested by being smoked.

Because of cocaine's high price it has always been considered the Cadillac of drugs. A gram, or less than one-thirtieth an ounce, of the drug currently sells for between $50 and $120. Such an amount can easily be consumed in a single evening by one or two relatively new users. Cocaine's cost has resulted in an association between its use and people of glamour and wealth. This image has no doubt been partly responsible for the increase in the drug's popularity during

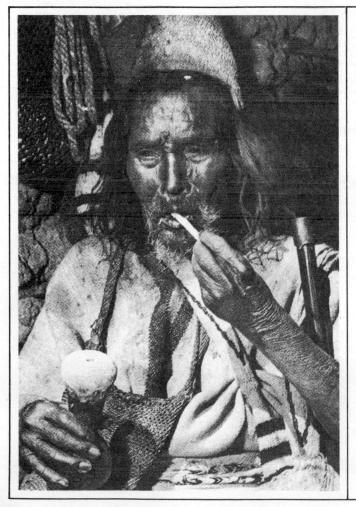

A Peruvian Indian adds lime to the coca quid packed between his cheek and gum to facilitate the drug's absorption through the membranes of the mouth. The ancient practice of chewing coca leaves remains the most common method of ingesting cocaine among Indians living in the Andes mountains.

the 1970s and especially since 1976. Today, despite the cost, the use of cocaine pervades all economic levels of society. Though the number of first-time cocaine users has leveled off, cocaine's increased availability has contributed to a rise in frequency and quantity of use per person. As a result, more people are experiencing cocaine-related problems and seeking treatment for them. Unfortunately, adequate treatment methods and facilities are not always readily available. This situation has resulted in a sense of urgency being felt toward the problem of cocaine abuse across the nation.

How Cocaine Is Ingested

Despite reports to the contrary, cocaine is readily absorbed into the bloodstream when taken orally. Coca leaves were chewed by Indians living in the Andes mountains in ancient times, and this is still the most prevalent method of cocaine use there. A major reason for the Peruvian Indian use of this drug is to help combat fatigue and hunger. Because the effects are not long lasting (1 to 2 hours when chewed), Indians store the masticated leaves in their cheeks so that low concentrations of cocaine are released throughout the day. When leaves are chewed, cocaine is absorbed from the membranes of the mouth and, since some is inadvertently swallowed, from the stomach and intestines. Peruvian Indians combine lime or ash with the coca leaves to facilitate the drug's absorption.

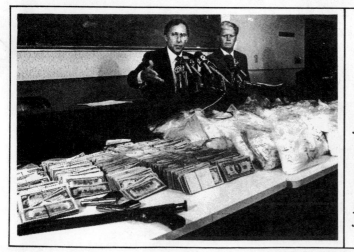

Los Angeles police display goods confiscated in a major cocaine bust—$402,000 in cash, 3 handguns, and 87 pounds of cocaine. Although federal drug enforcement efforts against cocaine have tripled since 1981, the illicit market remains strong and yields high profits for traffickers.

Outside of South America, cocaine is most frequently used in the form of a powder, which is readily absorbed from all mucous membranes such as those lining the mouth, nasal passages, and gastrointestinal tract. One reason why powder is the preferred form of use is that it is difficult to smuggle large quantities of coca leaves across national borders. Consequently, the cocaine problem in the United States involves cocaine hydrochloride, which has been extracted from coca leaves, illegally transported into the country, and sold on the black market. To increase profits, cocaine hydrochloride is diluted, or adulterated, with sugars and other drugs such as amphetamines and the much more inexpensive and more readily available local anesthetics. Thus, using street cocaine, which is only 12% to 75% pure, exposes the user to other unknown and potentially dangerous substances.

In the late 19th century cocaine was sometimes taken orally after being dissolved in elixirs and wine. These solutions were touted as miracle drugs that could cure all types

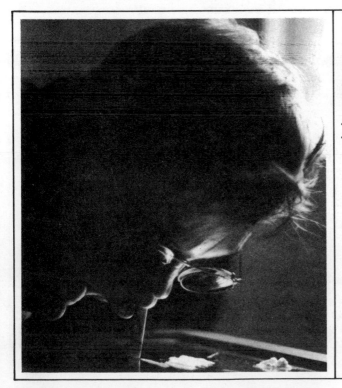

A person inhales "lines" of cocaine from a mirror. "Snorting" cocaine is the most popular means of taking the drug, although it is frequently responsible for severe nasal damage.

of ailments, reduce fatigue, and improve mood. Though cocaine can indeed produce its characteristic effects when ingested in solution, they are relatively minor compared to those produced when it is consumed in other ways.

The Intranasal Route

"Snorting," or the intranasal route, is the most popular way to take cocaine today. Generally, users purchase cocaine powder that is in the form of the hydrochloride. To prepare it for inhalation, the powder is finely chopped and the user inhales it through a tube.

Within seconds of sniffing, people report a numbing sensation in the nose and then a "freeze," which lasts approximately 5 minutes. There is then a gradual sense of mild exhilaration, euphoria, and increased energy. The "high" reaches a peak in 10 to 20 minutes and subsides almost completely within 60 minutes. The stimulatory effects last for 20 to 40 minutes. In an attempt to maintain their high, users often continue to snort at regular intervals, perhaps every 30 minutes or so, usually until their supply is gone.

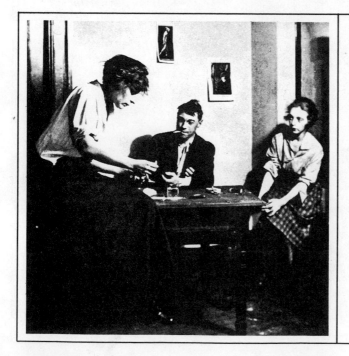

A photo from the 1930s depicts a small group of people preparing to "shoot up" cocaine. Injecting the drug intravenously can create serious problems, such as overdose and dangerous infections.

The Intravenous Route

Many frequent or more experienced cocaine users administer the drug intravenously. The usual dose is 10 mg. Although many of the physiological and subjective effects of the drug are the same as those produced by intranasal ingestion, by injecting the drug users often experience an intense "rush" within just a minute or two. This rush wears off within 30 minutes, and users often repeat the experience by injecting more of the drug if it is available. It has been shown experimentally and substantiated by street users' reports that a smaller dose is required when the intravenous route is used as compared to the intranasal route. In addition, intravenous users are more apt to go on a binge in order to reinstate the effects. As a result they do numerous lines until they or the supply of the drug are exhausted.

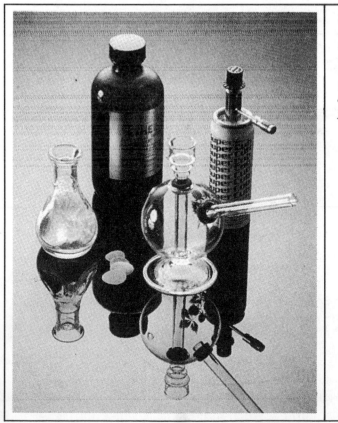

Freebasing, a process of purifying and then smoking cocaine with the paraphernalia shown here, is a highly dangerous form of cocaine abuse often preferred by addicts.

Smoking Cocaine

The smoking of coca paste is widespread in Peru, Ecuador, Colombia, and Bolivia, where this form of the drug is readily available. Among adolescent males of these countries this practice is considered to be epidemic. Compulsive coca-paste smoking, which includes the consumption of large amounts of the drug, is common. Peruvian users, for example, sometimes smoke up to 60 gm of coca paste in a single session.

The dried paste, which contains from 40% to 90% cocaine sulfate, is smoked in a cigarette in combination with tobacco or marijuana. The euphoria and central nervous system stimulation produced by smoking coca paste occur almost immediately because of the rapid absorption of cocaine from the lungs. However, the pleasant effects are relatively short-lived and, even though the concentration of the drug in the blood is still high, within a few minutes cocaine smokers become anxious, irritable, and depressed. To avoid this undesirable reaction users sometimes continue to smoke coca paste for several hours, though they rarely regain the initial euphoria. With continued smoking, hallucinations and psychotic behavior may develop. In addition, many of the impurities in coca paste, such as kerosene, can produce their own toxic effects.

In 1985 coca paste is not being imported into the United States on a large-scale basis. This situation may change, however, since the paste, which requires only crude processing, is cheaper to produce than cocaine hydrochloride. On the other hand, the selling of coca paste may be less profitable to dealers. Cocaine hydrochloride is generally adulterated, which increases dealers' profits, but it is more difficult to do this with coca paste. Also, the paste is bulkier and thus more difficult to transport.

Freebasing, another form of cocaine smoking, is becoming increasingly popular in the United States. Cocaine hydrochloride is converted into a form suitable for freebasing by the chemical process described earlier.

The base of cocaine is smoked in a water pipe in a manner similar to the way marijuana is frequently smoked. Interestingly, because much of the cocaine is lost through condensation and escaped smoke, only 5% to 6% of the drug actually gets through the pipe. As a result, people must use large quantities of cocaine when freebasing. A single inhalation of the freebase requires approximately 100 mg, and users sometimes consume up to 30 gm or more in a 24-hour binge. Smoking freebase is the most expensive form of cocaine abuse.

Why then has freebasing become so popular? A major reason is that, like injecting cocaine intravenously, this method produces an intense rush. In fact, freebasing produces greater subjective feelings of vigor and pleasure than all the other methods of administration. It also produces a greater craving for another dose of cocaine than does cocaine administered intravenously. But freebasing is also the most harmful form of cocaine abuse. Several studies have shown that freebasing can damage the lungs, and complications may result from the burning of freebase because of the flammable solvents used in the extraction process. Explosions can even occur, as was the case in the much-publicized and nearly fatal incident involving comedian Richard Pryor.

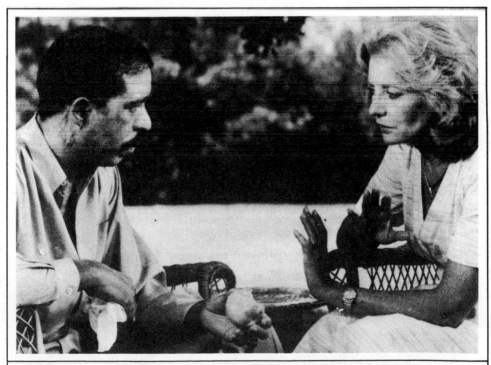

Richard Pryor, shown here in a 1980 interview with Barbara Walters, was severely burned when ether, a highly combustible substance used in the freebasing process, exploded in his face.

Anatomical drawing from the notebook of Italian Renaissance artist Leonardo da Vinci. The physiological effects of cocaine include an increase in respiration rate, blood pressure, and body temperature.

CHAPTER 2

THE EFFECTS OF COCAINE ON THE BODY

The nervous system can be seen as having two major divisions: the central nervous system (CNS), which includes the brain and spinal cord, and the peripheral nervous system (PNS), which is the system of neurons outside the CNS. However, since most actions and sensations involve both systems, this division is somewhat arbitrary. For example, when a person picks up an object, though the final neural event occurs in the periphery and involves a communication between a nerve and a muscle, the initiation and coordination of the act occur in specialized areas of the brain.

The nervous system is clearly involved in the control of motor function and the processing of incoming sensory events. However, there is also a specialized system responsible for maintaining bodily functions. This system is called the autonomic nervous system (ANS). The heart, lungs, and digestive system are controlled by the ANS. This control is accomplished by two entirely separate subdivisions—the sympathetic and parasympathetic systems—that have opposite effects on functioning. Most organs are innervated, or supplied, by the nerves of both systems. For instance, the sympathetic system increases cardiovascular activity, such as elevating heart rate, whereas the parasympathetic system reduces the heart's activity. In this way the body continually adjusts necessary functions with little or no voluntary intervention.

Cocaine as a Local Anesthetic

In July 1884 Sigmund Freud published an article on cocaine, at the end of which he alluded to the drug's potential use as a local anesthetic. The same year, excited by the article, ophthalmologist Carl Koller did an experiment and found that cocaine applied to the cornea of the eye produced an anesthesia strong enough to permit eye surgery. His findings, reported at a medical conference in Heidelberg, were considered a major medical breakthrough.

A local anesthetic produces a loss of sensation, including pain, in a specific area and does not depend on an interaction with the CNS. For instance, dentists give patients a local anesthetic, Novocaine, when performing what would otherwise be painful procedures. The numbing action is due to the drug's interference with nerve transmission to the brain.

When at rest, a nerve's outside surface is positively

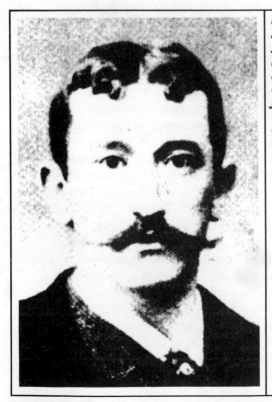

Carl Koller, the Austrian ophthalmologist and associate of Sigmund Freud who, in 1884, discovered that cocaine could be applied as a local anesthetic in eye surgery. Although Koller's findings were initially hailed as a medical breakthrough, the use of cocaine as a local anesthetic was eventually discontinued because it produced harmful side effects such as damage to the cornea.

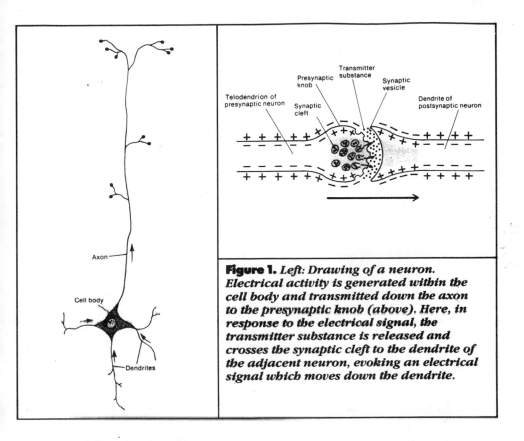

Figure 1. *Left: Drawing of a neuron. Electrical activity is generated within the cell body and transmitted down the axon to the presynaptic knob (above). Here, in response to the electrical signal, the transmitter substance is released and crosses the synaptic cleft to the dendrite of the adjacent neuron, evoking an electrical signal which moves down the dendrite.*

charged with sodium ions and its inside is negatively charged with potassium ions. When the nerve is stimulated, there is a localized rush of positive ions into the nerve axon (see Figure 1), which causes a change in its polarity. To compensate for this change, negatively charged potassium ions rush out. This localized change of polarity moves down the axon until it reaches the terminal. Between the terminal and the receptor of the adjacent nerve there is a space, or synaptic cleft, across which the nerve impulse cannot pass. However, when the impulse reaches the terminal a chemical, or neurotransmitter, is released. The neurotransmitter crosses the synapse and stimulates the receptor, thus creating a new electrical impulse. In order to "feel" a sensation such as pain, information has to be transmitted from one neuron to another until it reaches the brain, where it is processed and finally interpreted as a sensation of pain. It is only then that the individual is aware of feeling pain.

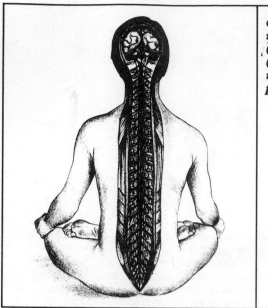

Cocaine raises the levels of the neurotransmitter norepinephrine (NE) in the central nervous system (illustrated here), causing an increase in heart rate and physical activity.

Cocaine produces its anesthetic effects by interfering with the transmission of information. Specifically, the drug inhibits the exchange of sodium and potassium in the nerve fibers, and thus the impulse is not able to move along the neuron. As a result, communication between neurons is impossible.

Although cocaine was originally used as a local anesthetic in eye surgery, it was soon found to produce unwanted side effects such as damage to the cornea. Because of this, other local anesthetics were synthesized that neither produced cocaine's toxic effects nor possessed its potential for abuse.

In contrast to other local anesthetics, cocaine also is a potent vasoconstrictor. This means that it narrows, or constricts, blood vessels. This property makes the drug useful in surgical procedures involving the upper passages of the respiratory tract, where excessive bleeding can be especially dangerous. Furthermore, cocaine has a prolonged anesthetic action that allows long and painful surgery of the nose to be easily performed.

In addition to its local anesthetic and vasoconstrictive actions, cocaine also increases the effects of the neurotransmitters responsible for activating the sympathetic nervous system. This property helps to explain many of cocaine's actions, both in the body's peripheral areas and in the brain. Activated sympathetic neurons release the neurotransmitter norepinephrine (NE), which works upon specialized receptors of other neurons, thereby activating them. The effect of NE on the receptors is stopped by a mechanism that essentially pumps the neurotransmitter back into the nerve cell from which it was first released. Cocaine, however, blocks this pumping action. Consequently, the stimulatory effects of NE are enhanced because there is more NE present at the receptor site for a longer time.

Cocaine has an effect wherever NE acts as a neurotransmitter. One of the most important systems of the body affected by cocaine is the cardiovascular system. Moderate doses of the drug increase heart rate and blood pressure. The increased heart rate is a result of the increased levels of NE and epinephrine (another neurotransmitter) acting directly on the heart. The increased blood pressure is due to the vasoconstrictive action of cocaine. Since the extent of the effects depends on the size of the dose, large quantities of cocaine ingested by any route of administration can result in death from cardiac failure.

The Effects of Cocaine in the Brain

Cocaine's exact mechanism of action in the brain or central nervous system is not completely known. As in the sympathetic system, NE is also a neurotransmitter in the brain, and its effects are enhanced by cocaine's ability to block the mechanism that pumps NE back into the nerve. Cocaine also blocks the reuptake of other brain neurotransmitters such as dopamine. Because of these CNS effects, cocaine is classified as a psychomotor stimulant.

In animals, cocaine, as well as other stimulants, produces a dose-related effect on motor behavior. In mice and rats, low doses of amphetamine enhance exploration, grooming, rearing, and general locomotion. At moderate doses, these activities disappear and are replaced by stereotypy, or behavior repeated without variation, such as gnawing, sniffing, and licking. As the dose is increased even further, convulsions, coma, and death result. Based on what is known about the neurochemical actions of psychomotor stimulants in general, it is thought that the increased locomotor activity is controlled by systems that use both NE and dopamine. The dopaminergic system is presumed to control the stereotypy.

Another action of psychomotor stimulant drugs is a reduction in both food and water intake. However, this could be a result of the general increase in activity produced by stimulants and not because of their direct effect on appetite. In addition, the presence of stereotypic behavior could actually interfere with the ability of an organism to eat or drink. Therefore, one cannot conclude that these animals are not hungry or thirsty—they just do not participate in these activities when given amphetamine or cocaine.

An increase in aggressive behavior has been demonstrated in a variety of species following doses of amphetamine that do not produce stereotypy. However, despite the fact that amphetamine produces an increase in aggressive behavior, cocaine has been shown only to reduce aggression.

Cocaine also increases respiration rate and body temperature, and induces vomiting by stimulating the center of the brain controlling nausea. At high doses, tremors and convulsions may result. These stimulatory effects can rapidly lead to a collapse of the central nervous system, which may lead to respiratory failure and/or cardiac arrest and finally death.

Cocaine's effects on the brain can be seen by measuring

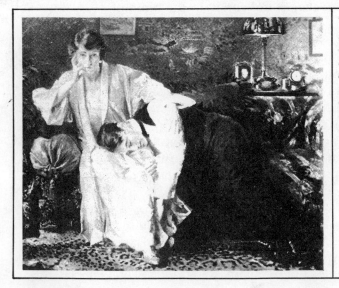

"Cocaine," a 19th-century painting by Alfred Priest, depicts the fatigue, depression, and general lack of motivation that often occur after the initial euphoria of a cocaine dose subsides.

and comparing the electrical activity of the brain before and after drug administration. This type of activity can be monitored by an electroencephalograph (EEG), which records the brain's electrical impulses through electrodes placed on the scalp. An injection of cocaine produces an increase in electrical activity in the limbic system and a structure called the amygdala, areas of the brain thought to be associated with mood, emotion, and feelings of pleasure.

After repeated exposure to cocaine, certain areas in the limbic system are more susceptible to a type of seizure activity that resembles an epileptic fit. Because of this, it is possible that by studying the mechanism of cocaine's progressively increasing effects on EEG arousal one may gain an understanding of epilepsy. For instance, the increased EEG activity produced by cocaine (as well as other local anesthetics) is similar to that produced by what is called *kindling*, an enhanced behavioral and electrophysiological response to low levels of repeated electrical stimulation of the brain. By using kindling, electrical stimuli previously incapable of inducing seizures have produced behavioral convulsions. Since cocaine and amphetamine both induce similar EEG activity patterns, as well as convulsions, one theory is that kindling is responsible for the supersensitivity and toxic psychosis that can result from repeated doses of these CNS stimulants.

The Psychological Effects of Cocaine

Depression, euphoria, and anger have a physiological basis. For example, electrical stimulation of certain areas of the brain produces feelings of pleasure. Although researchers do not yet completely understand how small changes in neurotransmitters translate into changes in a person's psychological state, there is little question that any drug that alters the functioning of the brain will have psychological effects. In fact, it is usually these effects that attract drug abusers.

The psychological effects of cocaine are complex and are influenced by the environment, the dose, the route of administration, and the characteristics and experience of the user. The major effect sought by most recreational users is what is frequently termed "euphoria." In addition, users describe an intense rush that is experienced when cocaine is smoked or injected. People report feelings of increased mental alertness, sexual desire, and sensory awareness and are more energetic, talkative, and self-confident. Cocaine also causes a profound decrease in appetite, which in a chronic user can result in severe weight loss as well as a nutritional imbalance. Finally, use of this drug results in loss of sleep.

With continual use of cocaine, the high is frequently unobtainable and, in fact, may be replaced by feelings of dysphoria and displeasure. Shortly after the first high many users "crash," or experience sleepiness, irritability, feelings of depression, and lack of motivation. In those individuals who smoke, these undesirable effects occur within seconds after the initial euphoria. Because of this, users often increase their intake and/or repeatedly ingest the drug with the hope that they will be able to regain the initial pleasant feelings. With repeated use a psychosis similar to that produced by chronic high doses of amphetamine can replace the euphoria. In fact, the psychoses produced by both these drugs so closely resemble schizophrenia that physicians often have difficulty distinguishing between a drug-induced condition and a true psychiatric disorder.

The symptoms of cocaine psychosis usually include paranoia, delusions of persecution, and visual, auditory, and tactile hallucinations. Frequently the tactile hallucinations involve the sensation of insects crawling under the skin—a condition known as formication. In humans, the progressive increase in irritability, restlessness, paranoia, and suspiciousness associated with prolonged high-dose use may be a result of kindling.

How Unique Is Cocaine?

Cocaine has effects very similar to other CNS stimulants such as amphetamines (Benzedrine, Dexedrine). When administered intravenously, amphetamine produces euphoria, insomnia, reduced appetite, and the perception of enhanced physical strength. This drug is also administered in "runs" when injected, and the momentary rush is common. In fact, amphetamine addicts are unable to distinguish between the cocaine and the amphetamine euphoria. In an experimental situation, subjects were unable to detect any difference between 8 mg to 16 mg of cocaine and 10 mg of amphetamine when the drugs were given intravenously. However, because amphetamine is longer lasting than cocaine, as time passes the drugs can be distinguished from each other.

When either amphetamine or cocaine ceases to be available, heavy users experience feelings of drug craving and their sleep becomes prolonged, their appetite returns, and feelings of fatigue and depression occur. However, it has not been scientifically demonstrated that a state of physical dependence is produced by either cocaine or amphetamine. Physical dependence is the adaptation of the body to the presence of a drug, such that when drug use is discontinued withdrawal symptoms appear which can be immediately alleviated by readministering the drug. Whether or not such a state is produced by stimulants is still a much-debated question.

In summary, cocaine, amphetamine, and other related CNS stimulants share similar behavioral, subjective, pharmacological, and toxic effects. However, it is presumed that cocaine's subjective effects and abuse potential are more intense, though this is difficult to prove.

The present cocaine epidemic may be due to its relative availability. When amphetamine was first synthesized in the 1930s, cocaine use was low. However, because of the spread of amphetamine abuse, in 1972 the prescribing and manufacturing of this drug was put under tighter control. Interestingly, the cocaine epidemic of the 1980s may in part be a result of the rescheduling and consequent decreased availability of amphetamine.

The Toxic Effects of Cocaine

Under a variety of circumstances cocaine can be lethal. For instance, some individuals are born lacking pseudocholinesterases, the enzymes necessary for the metabolism, or breakdown, of cocaine in the blood. Because of this, even a dose as low as 20 mg can cause death. However, individuals afflicted with this condition are rare.

More commonly, death results from much higher doses than 20 mg. Massive cocaine intoxication is characterized by CNS stimulation (restlessness, tremors, and convulsions) followed by depression (respiratory and cardiovascular failure). Because of increased demand on the heart during cocaine use, people with heart problems, such as hypertension or cardiovascular disease, are more prone to a fatal reaction. There are also rare cases of cerebral hemorrhages (a great discharge of blood in the brain) occurring from acute increases in blood pressure.

Sudden death from a massive overdose can also occur when cocaine is smuggled in various cavities of the body, a method called "body packing." Sometimes balloons, condoms, or plastic bags are filled with cocaine and swallowed by smugglers. These packets sometimes break, resulting in the absorption of excessive amounts of the drug and a massive overdose. Since many of the packets are made of semipermeable materials, even when the packets remain intact the cocaine can be absorbed into the body and cause death.

Some of cocaine's actions, such as vasoconstriction, increased physical activity, and stimulation of the heat-regulating center in the brain, lead to hyperthermia, or an increase in body temperature. This can be life threatening since proper cellular functioning throughout the body depends on normal temperature. At extreme internal temperatures, cells in the brain and the rest of the body die.

As previously described, cocaine alters the normal electrical activity of the brain. This can result in seizures or convulsive activity very similar to epilepsy. An overdose of cocaine can induce repeated convulsions that, unless emer-

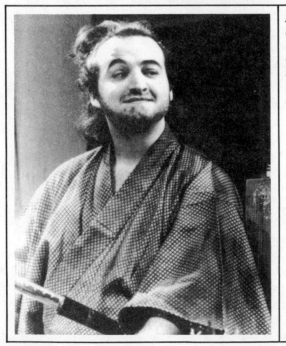

Mixing cocaine with other drugs can produce extremely unpredictable, sometimes fatal consequences. Comedian John Belushi died in 1982 from "speedballing," which involves ingesting a combination of heroin and cocaine.

gency measures are immediately taken, eventually lead to death. People who are taking medication to control epilepsy are more prone to seizures following cocaine administration.

Cocaine can also lead to death indirectly. For example, if the drug is taken intravenously, unsterile syringes can cause infections or disease. These infections can include hepatitis B, septicemia (blood poisoning), subacute bacterial endocarditis (the inflammation of the lining of the heart and its valves), and even incurable, fatal diseases such as AIDS (acquired immune deficiency syndrome). These infections occur because most drug abusers do not understand that a failure to use sterile techniques can result in the introduction of infection- or disease-producing agents into the body. Even if they do understand, sterile syringes and needles are difficult to obtain, since these items are only available with a doctor's prescription. Finally, in the drug culture, users are apt to share drugs and even syringes with friends. Because of this practice, diseases are easily transmitted.

The use of cocaine is closely connected to many other social problems. Accidents, particularly automobile accidents, are more likely to occur to individuals under the influence of cocaine. The post-cocaine depression, which can lead to suicidal and paranoid thoughts, may also result in violent behavior, including homicide. Furthermore, the illicit cocaine trade engenders a great deal of violence. Only recently, in retaliation for large seizures of cocaine by U.S. Drug Enforcement Agency officials, two drug enforcement agents were kidnapped in Mexico by drug traffickers and murdered.

Drug Interactions

When taken together, two or more drugs may produce effects that are greater than (synergistic), less than, or unrelated to the effects of any of the drugs alone. However, the effects of these combinations are often difficult to predict. Many cocaine users, and drug users in general, take other drugs in combination with cocaine. These may include alcohol, marijuana, barbiturates, tranquilizers, and methaqualone (Quaaludes). As a result of these combinations, serious toxicity (poisonous effects) can result. One example is the heroin/cocaine combination, known as "speedballing." Although the pleasurable effects of this combination have been touted, it can be lethal, as was the case with comedian John Belushi.

Drug combinations can also be ingested inadvertently. Street cocaine is frequently adulterated with substances such as sugar (to increase volume), other local anesthetics, and various CNS stimulants. Unfortunately, drug dealers are not generally knowledgeable or concerned about drug interactions, and drug buyers can never be sure of what they are purchasing. Thus, there is always the possibility of ingesting a dangerous combination.

Tolerance

One of the consequences of taking any drug repeatedly is tolerance. When this has occurred a person must take higher doses of the drug to achieve the level of effects experienced previously. In other words, with repeated administration there is a decreased responsiveness to the drug's effects. Tolerance may not develop to all of a drug's effects or to any of them at the same time. In addition, in some instances, reverse tolerance, or sensitization, develops. When this has occurred an organism becomes *more* sensitive to certain of the drug's effects.

Unfortunately, not much is known about tolerance to cocaine. However, a great deal of information is available on the ability of amphetamine to produce tolerance. Since these two drugs are similar, understanding amphetamine tolerance may be useful for predicting patterns of tolerance to cocaine.

Tolerance develops to some of amphetamine's effects on the central nervous system, including its euphoric, anorectic (appetite suppressant), and hyperthermic actions. Among chronic amphetamine users, an increase in dose is often needed to obtain the desired psychological effect. At the same time, there is an increased sensitivity to other effects on the central nervous system. For instance, individuals who have experienced the toxic psychosis induced by chronic high doses of amphetamine often experience these same adverse effects at lower doses if they resume amphetamine use.

Some animal studies have demonstrated the development of tolerance to cocaine's effects. With repeated administration, the initial decrease in food intake caused by this drug disappears. Cross-tolerance (a condition in which tolerance to one drug results in tolerance to another drug) to the appetite-suppressing effect has been demonstrated between amphetamine and cocaine in rats. However, after discontinuing use, tolerance to cocaine's anorectic effects rapidly disappears. In contrast, tolerance to amphetamine's effects on food consumption may last up to 45 days after termination of chronic use.

In experiments using human volunteers who were given repeated intravenous doses of cocaine, short-term tolerance developed to the cardiovascular and subjective effects. These effects were reduced even though blood levels of the drug continued to rise as injections continued. However, tolerance had completely disappeared by the next day.

As with amphetamine, there is some evidence that following repeated use reverse tolerance occurs to some of cocaine's CNS effects. In one study, animals receiving chronic administration of cocaine did not demonstrate any tolerance but instead became more sensitive. This was characterized by hyperactivity, increased body temperature, and, most importantly, a decrease in the dose of cocaine that would produce convulsions and death. Another study found that chronic cocaine use produced an enhancement of the behavioral and EEG responses in rats, including a sensitivity to cocaine's ability to induce convulsions.

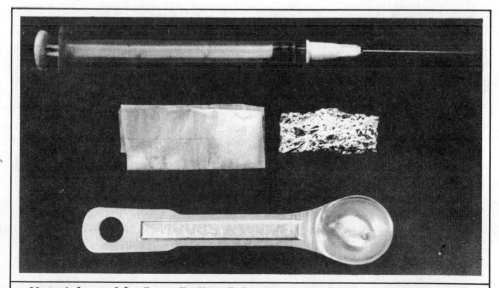

Materials used for "speedballing," the potentially fatal combination of cocaine and heroin: a hypodermic needle to inject the heroin, packets of both drugs, and a spoon used to prepare the drugs for injection.

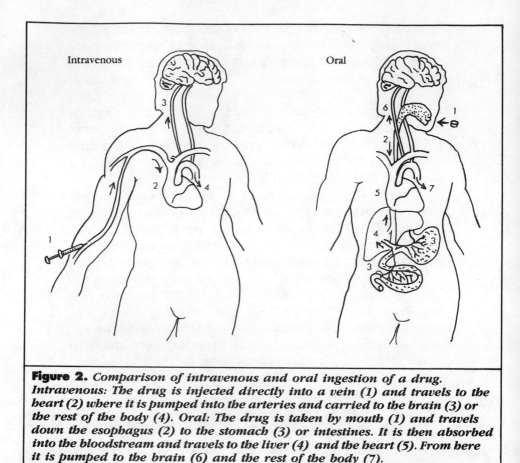

Figure 2. *Comparison of intravenous and oral ingestion of a drug. Intravenous: The drug is injected directly into a vein (1) and travels to the heart (2) where it is pumped into the arteries and carried to the brain (3) or the rest of the body (4). Oral: The drug is taken by mouth (1) and travels down the esophagus (2) to the stomach (3) or intestines. It is then absorbed into the bloodstream and travels to the liver (4) and the heart (5). From here it is pumped to the brain (6) and the rest of the body (7).*

Despite the fact that several studies report that the effects described above are increased by cocaine's repeated administration, there are other studies indicating that tolerance develops to these same effects. Some researchers have found that in rhesus monkeys given daily cocaine injections, the dose required to induce convulsions increased. The marked increase in heart rate and respiration rate was also reduced by daily cocaine injections. Furthermore, it has been demonstrated that tolerance develops rapidly to the stereotypic behavior induced by amphetamine. It remains for future research to determine the conditions under which repeated cocaine or amphetamine administration produces tolerance or increased sensitivity to these effects.

Little is known about tolerance to cocaine's euphoric effects. There is anecdotal evidence that with chronic use it becomes more difficult to obtain the desired high. In addition, increasing the dose or frequency may not reinstate these pleasurable effects. Consequently, increased use is not necessarily a response to tolerance to cocaine's effects.

Physical Dependence

Physical dependence is an adaptation of the body to the presence of a drug, such that the drug's absence produces withdrawal symptoms. The withdrawal syndrome produced by opiates such as heroin is a classic example. It is characterized by increased salivation, vomiting, restlessness, tremors, sweating, chills, diarrhea, and severe cramps. Barbiturate withdrawal includes similar symptoms, and, additionally, convulsions and even death. However, it is often difficult to distinguish between true physical dependence, which involves a physiological adaptation of the body, and the harmful effects produced by excessive drug use. Because body tissues adapt to the constant presence of a drug (tolerance), a person dependent on an opiate may appear to function normally until the drug is taken away.

For example, one of the effects of heroin is to decrease the rate of respiration. To maintain healthy functioning, the body responds to the presence of the drug and increases the breathing rate until the person appears normal. However, when the drug is taken away, the abnormal, *increased* respiration is revealed. Normal levels can be achieved immediately by once again ingesting the opiate.

In contrast, other drugs can produce toxic effects that do not disappear when drug use is discontinued. If more of the drug is given, these symptoms may get even worse. Therefore, illness following drug removal does not prove the existence of physical dependence unless the symptoms can be reversed by the administration of more drug.

There is general agreement among the scientific community that because there is no clear withdrawal syndrome following discontinuation of cocaine use, this drug does not produce physical dependence. However, persons who stop using cocaine do complain of depression, fatigue, agitation, sweating, chills, social withdrawal, drug craving, and eating and sleeping disturbances. However, these symptoms could be associated with a psychological dependence as well as with toxic reactions. In fact, many of these same complaints persist even with continued drug use. Clearly, more research is needed to verify the connection between these symptoms and physical dependence.

Though cocaine may not have dependence-producing properties common to the opiates and barbiturates, this does not mean that cocaine is less dangerous. Unfortunately, it is this lack of a true withdrawal syndrome that has led people to believe mistakenly that cocaine is a safe, recreational drug. The considerable amount of drug-seeking and drug-craving behavior observed in cocaine users who do not have access to the drug indicates, at least, a high level of psychological dependence. And, as mentioned previously, despite the fact that continued use may not necessarily reduce the undesirable effects, as long as the drug is available heavy users find it difficult to abstain from using cocaine.

Adverse Physical Effects from Chronic Use

The emergence of adverse reactions to cocaine appears to be dependent on the pattern of use. Compulsive and chronic users are more likely to enter treatment centers to receive both medical and psychiatric attention. As both dosage and frequency of cocaine use increase, adverse reactions (physical, psychological, and social) become present among all classes of users.

A toll-free hotline (800-COCAINE) established in 1983 enables anyone to call anonymously from anywhere in the United States 24 hours a day, seven days a week. People can call to seek advice and/or to ask for information or referrals for treatment. During one period callers were asked if they would participate in a confidential 20- to 30-minute telephone interview. Researchers used a random sample of 500 such callers to obtain information regarding the extent of the cocaine problem, the type of people who use cocaine (see also Chapter 3), and any adverse effects related to cocaine use.

Among these individuals, the most common physical complaints included fatigue, seizures, nausea, vomiting, chronic insomnia, severe headaches, nasal problems, and reduced sexual performance. Restlessness, irritability, and attentional or perceptual difficulties were also frequently reported. Over 80% of these people seeking help were intranasal users, dispelling the myth that this form of administration is safe and free of complications. Data from many sources indicate that smoking either the cocaine paste or freebase appears to produce even more severe physical complications, such as bronchitis, persistent coughing, blurred vision, and pulmonary dysfunction (circulation problems).

Psychosocial Problems

Chronic and compulsive cocaine use also leads to adverse psychological and social consequences. For instance, not infrequently job performance suffers and interpersonal relationships disintegrate. In addition, because of the drug's high cost, chronic use produces a tremendous financial burden. Many individuals have lost lucrative businesses as well as their

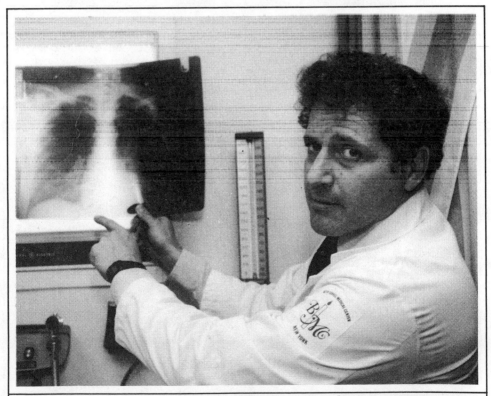

A doctor displays an x-ray indicating pneumonia, a disease common among abusers of cocaine. Recent evidence also strongly supports a link between regular cocaine use and heart disease.

homes and automobiles. And finally, to maintain their habit many cocaine abusers are forced to engage in illegal activities, such as stealing from an employer or family member and/or dealing in the black market.

Continued use can also result in other types of problems. Depression, anxiety, and irritability are the most frequent psychological complaints. Other psychological problems include difficulties in concentration and a loss of interest in friends and activities that are not drug related. Initially, many people use cocaine to enhance sociability and to increase sexual arousal. However, more than 50% of the people calling the cocaine hotline reported that they usually used cocaine when alone. Paradoxically, while increased sexual arousal is often given as a reason for continued cocaine use, the loss of sex drive and the inability to perform sexually are also major complaints of chronic cocaine users.

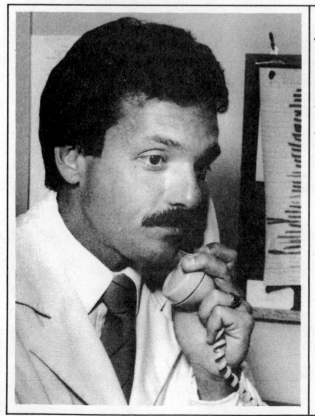

In 1983 Dr. Mark Gold founded a 24-hour toll-free hotline (800—COCAINE) to provide advice, information, and treatment referrals for people suffering from either physical or psychological problems related to cocaine abuse.

Unfortunately, since the desirable effects of cocaine diminish with continued and chronic use and are replaced by adverse effects, users often try to alleviate the unpleasant effects by increasing their cocaine use to a point where they lose control. They exhibit a persistent craving and compulsion to use cocaine despite the serious negative consequences and the relative rarity of positive effects. Cocaine becomes a way of life such that the user becomes preoccupied with obtaining and taking the drug. Of those who called the hotline, the majority (83%) said they could not resist cocaine when it was available. They believed they had become addicted to the drug and had lost control of their lives. Bingeing, or using cocaine continually for more than 24 hours, was common. Many said that cocaine was more important than food, sex, or even friends and family. Although the people calling knew that cocaine was having adverse

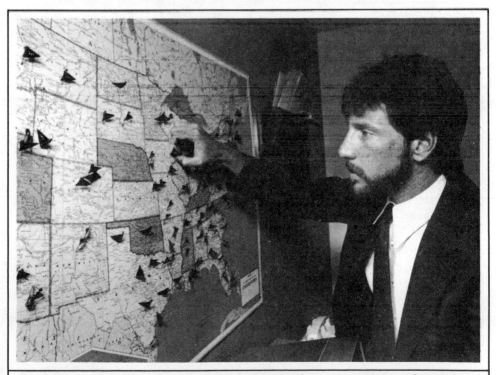

A worker at 800–COCAINE points to a map used in connection with a survey of cocaine abusers, 83% of whom admitted to psychological dependency and a craving for the drug despite its negative effects.

effects on their psychological well-being, their social and interpersonal relationships, and their career, their major concern was how to alleviate the undesirable physical effects.

Cocaine and the Law

Under federal law cocaine is still defined as a narcotic, even though it is not an opiate but a stimulant. This classification has a historical basis. In 1914 the Harrison Narcotics Act was passed to restrict the use and manufacture of drugs of abuse. These included cocaine as well as true narcotics such as morphine, but no distinctions as to the drug's different pharmacological effects were made. As a result, any drug considered dangerous at that time was called a narcotic, a mistake that still is commonly made.

In 1970 the Controlled Substances Act was passed by the U.S. Congress to provide a means for legal control of psychoactive drugs. Under the joint control of the Food and Drug Administration (FDA) and the Drug Enforcement Administration (DEA), drugs are placed into one of five schedules according to their potential for abuse. These designations are based upon what is known about a drug's actual abuse and, particularly in the case of new drugs, the similarity of its pharmacological actions to the actions of known drugs of abuse. Each of these schedules establishes how drugs will be distributed by manufacturers and monitored by pharmacists and physicians. The schedules also specify the maximum penalties for illegal possession and distribution of drugs in the category. Schedule I drugs, considered to have a high abuse potential and no therapeutic application, have the most severe restrictions and penalties. Drugs in Schedule II also have a high abuse potential but in addition have therapeutic benefits. Drugs in Schedules III through V are considered to have correspondingly less abuse potential and greater therapeutic usefulness.

Today most narcotics, amphetamines, and cocaine are controlled under Schedule II of the Controlled Substances Act. Though cocaine has a high abuse potential, it is still useful for certain types of surgery as a local anesthetic. Because cocaine is a Schedule II drug, possession by a first offender is punishable by a term of imprisonment of not more than one year, a fine of not more than $5,000, or both. For additional offenses, these penalties are drastically increased. Trafficking in cocaine, considered to be a far more serious crime, is punishable by a maximum of 15 years' imprisonment, a maximum fine of $125,000, or both for first offenders. As with possession, these penalties increase dramatically with additional offenses. Of interest, these maximum penalties can be doubled if the offense occurs in, on, or within 1,000 feet of a public or private elementary or secondary school.

In addition to these federal laws, states have drug laws that are enforced by local authorities. Laws concerning possession of cocaine vary from state to state and also are dependent on the amount of the drug involved. For instance, in Alabama, penalties for first offenders possessing small quantities of cocaine can bring a prison sentence of anywhere from one month to 15 years. A first offense for trafficking cocaine can result in a fine of up to $25,000 in addition to a maximum of 15 years in prison.

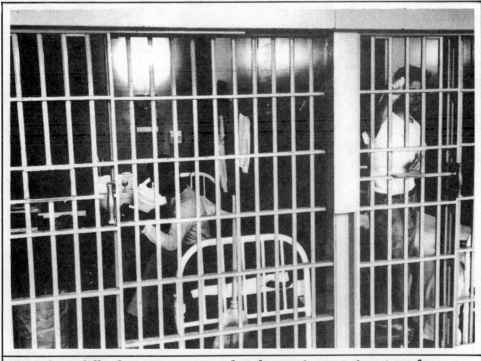

Drug laws differ from state to state, but the maximum prison term for first-time cocaine offenders varies from 1 year for possession to 15 years for dealing. Repeat offenders receive more severe penalties.

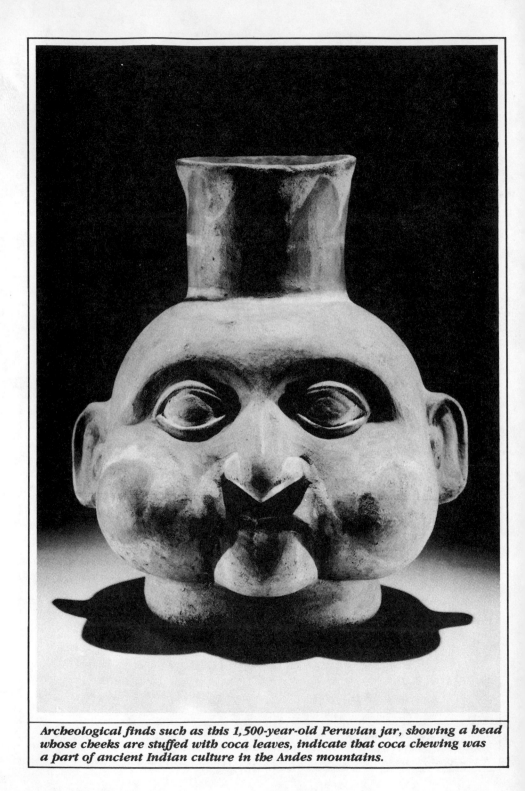

Archeological finds such as this 1,500-year-old Peruvian jar, showing a head whose cheeks are stuffed with coca leaves, indicate that coca chewing was a part of ancient Indian culture in the Andes mountains.

CHAPTER 3

COCAINE USE:
HISTORY, PATTERNS, TRENDS

Long before cocaine was extracted from the coca plant
(see Chapter 4), the leaves were chewed by the Indians of
Peru and other South American countries. This practice began
before recorded history, so our knowledge about this early
period is derived totally from archeological sources. Line
drawings on pottery found in many areas of northwestern
South America show evidence that coca chewing was part of
the culture even before the rise of the Incan Empire, perhaps
as early as 3000 B.C.E. (Before Common Era, equivalent to
B.C.), and that coca's effects on mood and behavior were
profound and much appreciated by the Indians.

The coca plant was considered a gift of the gods and was
used during religious rituals, burials, and for special purposes.
For instance, because there were no horses, the only way to
communicate between parts of the Empire was to send mes-
sages by runners. These runners traveled long distances in
the Andean highlands, where even walking is difficult because
of the reduced oxygen at such high altitudes. By chewing
the coca leaves, the runners were able to travel these long
distances rapidly even without food or water.

By the time the Spaniards arrived in the 16th century,
the Incan Empire was in decline. Interestingly, by this time
coca was no longer used only by the ruling class or only in

association with ritual. Although it still occupied an important place in the religious and cultural rituals of the Indians, there is evidence that many people used coca on a daily basis. At first the Spaniards attempted to prevent the Indians from using coca because they believed it was a barrier to their attempts to convert the native people to Christianity. However, it soon became apparent that by allowing the now enslaved Indians to use coca the Conquistadors could force them to do enormous amounts of work in the gold and silver mines despite the difficult conditions of the highlands. It even became a practice to pay the Indians coca leaves for their work. As a result, unlike during Incan times, the Spanish cultivated the coca plants and the use of the leaves became a part of daily life for many Indians.

Coca leaves, along with other natural psychoactive substances such as coffee, tea, and tobacco, were brought to Europe from South America by the explorers in the 16th century. But unlike these other substances, coca leaves remained unpopular until the 19th century. This unpopularity may have been due to the deterioration of the leaves during transport. Warm and humid conditions, such as those en-

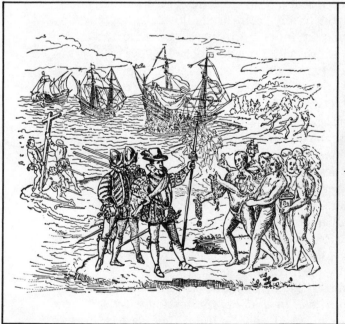

Francisco Pizarro, arriving in Peru, led the Spanish conquest of the Incan empire in the 16th century. After initially condemning coca chewing, the Conquistadors subsequently encouraged the practice among the enslaved Indians when it seemed to increase their work efforts in the gold and silver mines.

countered in the holds of ships during the long voyages from the New World, destroy the potency of the leaves. As a result, the effects of the imported coca leaves were minimal.

The Isolation of Cocaine

In 1855 the chemist Gaedecke made an extract from coca leaves and prepared a crystalline substance with an oily residue, which he named "erythroxyline." Seven years later, Albert Niemann, an assistant to Friedrich Wöhler, the "father of synthetic organic chemistry," extracted then purified cocaine. Although the chemical structure of cocaine was suggested at the end of the 19th century, it was not until 1955 that the chemical structure of cocaine was verified.

Not knowing the chemical structure of the extracted drug, however, did not prevent its use. After its purification by Niemann, the use and misuse of cocaine spread rapidly. Almost immediately, research on its effects in both animals and humans began. For example, in 1883 Theodor Aschenbrandt, an army surgeon, wrote extensively about cocaine's

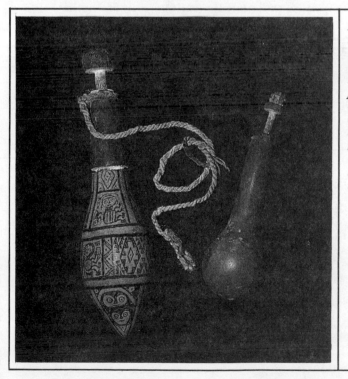

Lime gourds, like those pictured here, have long been used by South American Indians as part of the practice of coca chewing. By combining lime with coca leaves and holding them in their mouths, the Indians could prolong the effects of the drug.

usefulness in combatting battle fatigue and enabling wounded soldiers to function. His writing caught the attention of a young Viennese neurologist, Sigmund Freud. Until very recently, the most definitive description of the psychological and physiological effects of cocaine was contained in Freud's writings, most notably *Uber Coca*. Freud also conducted extensive experiments on the effects of cocaine on reaction times and muscular energy, as well as its effects on psychological mood. Often these experiments used only a single subject, Freud himself.

As a result of his findings, Freud believed strongly that cocaine was a miracle drug capable of curing a variety of ailments and making normal life more pleasant. In *Uber Coca*, Freud suggested that cocaine be used for a variety of therapeutic purposes, such as to increase a person's physical capacity during stressful times (e.g., in wartime, on long journeys, and for mountain climbing); to restore mental capacity decreased by fatigue; and to improve "psychic debilities" such as melancholia (the old term for depression). Freud also recommended cocaine for digestive disorders of the stomach, even those that merely resulted from eating too

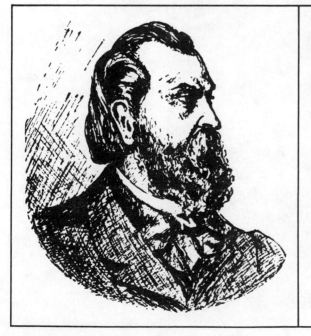

In 1862 Albert Niemann extracted a coca alkaloid that he named "cocaine." Extensive research into the drug's effects began soon after the discovery, but unfortunately cocaine later became widely abused.

large a meal, as well as for asthma and diseases thought to be due to tissue degeneration.

The list of the diseases Freud and many other prominent physicians at the time believed could be cured by cocaine is truly impressive and certainly contributed to the general feeling that cocaine could do just about anything, even cure syphilis. But the most unbelievable claim that was especially promoted by Freud was that cocaine could be given as a cure for morphine and alcohol addiction. Much of Freud's knowledge of this claim came from medical journal accounts and promotional brochures from pharmaceutical firms in the United States. One of the brochures stated that "in cocaine we have a remedy, whose physiological actions and therapeutic effects as recorded by competent observers, leave no doubt as to its great efficacy in the treatment of the alcoholic habit, its most specific action in affording relief to the victims of the opium habit." Freud also firmly believed and stated that "the treatment of morphine addiction with coca does

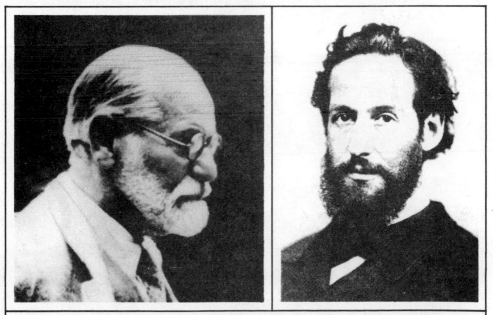

Sigmund Freud (left), who initially advocated the therapeutic use of cocaine, prescribed the drug as a cure for the morphine addiction of Ernst von Fleischl-Marxow (right). Tragically, Fleischl-Marxow became addicted to both drugs and later died of morphine poisoning.

not, therefore, result merely in the exchange of one kind of addiction for another—it does not turn the morphine addict into a *coquero*; the use of coca is only temporary."

In part because of Freud's writings and his excessive view of the benefits of cocaine, its use spread. The drug was available in Europe and the United States in a variety of preparations, including tonics and patent medicines. One of the most famous was a coca-containing wine marketed as Vin Mariani, whose advertisements included testimonials to the glories of the wine from popes, monarchs, U.S. presidents, and famous people such as Jules Verne and Thomas Edison. Another famous beverage that contained cocaine was Coca-Cola, which was advertised as "the brain tonic and intellectual soda-fountain beverage." Although caffeine has replaced cocaine in "Coke," even today it is flavored by decocainized coca leaves.

Although cocaine was highly regarded in the 1880s and 1890s, by the turn of the century its potential for abuse was beginning to be realized. One of the most tragic examples involved a close friend of Freud's, Ernst von Fleischl-Marxow, who was addicted to morphine. When Freud treated his condition with cocaine, Fleischl-Marxow quickly became heavily

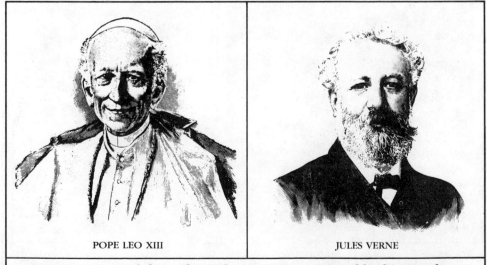

POPE LEO XIII

JULES VERNE

Pope Leo XIII and the author Jules Verne were two public figures who endorsed Vin Mariani, a highly popular mixture of wine and coca leaves that became available in 1865.

involved with the drug and began to use it excessively. Within a year he was taking so much cocaine that he suffered toxic psychosis and later died. Although Freud may not have ceased his own use of cocaine for several years, he and others began to write about the drug's horrors. One scientist of the time pronounced that cocaine was "the third scourge of humanity" (after alcohol and opium).

There was also a growing belief in the United States that the use of cocaine by blacks gave them superhuman powers. There are reports that law enforcement officers in the South switched to high caliber guns to protect themselves from the supposed menace of cocaine-using blacks on the rampage. This fear of minorities plus the increasing knowledge of cocaine's abuse led many state governments to restrict the use of cocaine. Thus, in 1914 the federal Harrison Narcotics Act prohibited the use of this drug in patent medicines and made the recreational use of cocaine illegal, as it remains today. As a result of these measures, the manufacture, distribution, and use of cocaine became strictly regulated. From the 1930s to the late 1960s, except among such individuals as entertainers and jazz musicians, the abuse of cocaine was largely non-existent.

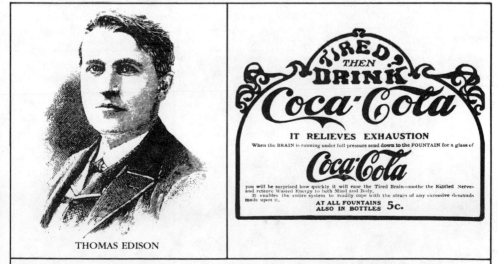

THOMAS EDISON

American inventor Thomas Edison also endorsed Vin Mariani. In 1888 Coca-Cola, which initially contained cocaine, advertised itself as "the drink that relieves exhaustion."

One can only speculate on the reasons for this decrease in use, but there are some reasonable explanations. In 1932 amphetamine, a potent psychomotor stimulant with cocaine-like properties, was synthesized, and it appears that this drug replaced cocaine as a recreational drug. Amphetamine, which had longer-lasting effects than cocaine, was inexpensive and widely available from physicians as a weight-reducing drug. But amphetamine's usefulness in the treatment of obesity was marginal and, in addition, serious adverse effects, such as brain damage, had become associated with its use. Therefore, when the extent of its abuse was finally appreciated, its availability was restricted. In 1972 the FDA made amphetamine a Schedule II drug, which forced closer monitoring of its production and distribution. After this time amphetamine was viewed as a potentially dangerous drug and it was no longer readily prescribed by physicians.

Cocaine in the 1970s

At the same time that the evils of amphetamine were being stressed, there were reports that cocaine did not have significant toxic effects. Few deaths from cocaine overdoses were confirmed and it seemed that few cocaine users ever sought medical help or treatment. As a result, many people made the erroneous conclusion that cocaine was a safe drug. The report from the National Commission on Marijuana and

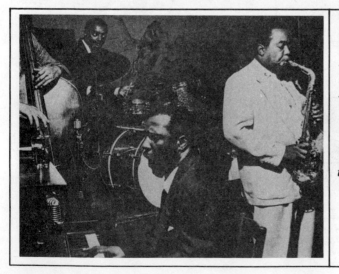

With the exception of some jazz musicians and entertainers, such as Charlie Parker (on sax), most people in the United States refrained from taking cocaine after the Harrison Narcotics Act outlawed recreational use of the drug in 1914.

Drug Abuse in 1973 stated that little social cost related to cocaine had been verified in the United States. Because of amphetamine's bad publicity, which was rightly deserved, and the reports that cocaine appeared to lack amphetamine's toxicity despite its similar effects, in the 1970s cocaine was rediscovered as a recreational drug. However, the potential for cocaine abuse was predicted by many experts. Doctors D. R. Wesson and D. E. Smith said: "If the drug were more readily available at a substantially lower cost, or if socio-cultural rituals endorsed and supported the higher dose patterns, more destructive patterns of abuse could develop."

In the early 1970s cocaine abuse had not yet become a major problem. The intranasal route was used almost exclusively and there was a low incidence of chronic use and no confirmed evidence of deaths due to cocaine overdoses. Since then the pattern of cocaine abuse has changed dramatically.

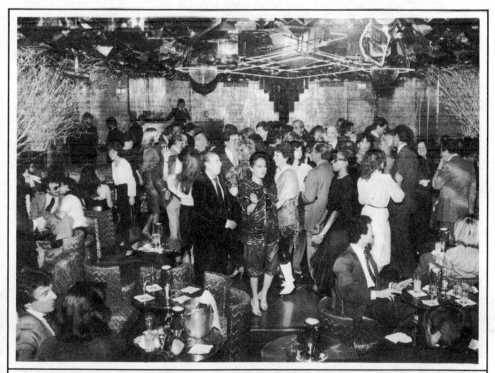

Cocaine came back into fashion in the 1970s. The drug's surge in popularity, particularly in nightclubs and discotheques, can be partly attributed to the chic exclusivity implicit in its high price.

An Epidemic of the 1980s

Reports from the National Household Survey sponsored by the National Institute on Drug Abuse indicate that those who have tried cocaine at least once rose from 5.4 million in 1974 to 21.6 million in 1982—a four-fold increase. In 1977 there were approximately 1.6 million regular users (defined as persons using cocaine at least once per month) compared to 4.3 million in 1979. This number of regular users remained constant through 1982.

The demand for treatment and the incidence of medical crises associated with cocaine use have also increased dramatically since 1976. Data reflecting the incidence of adverse cocaine-related consequences are collected by the Drug Abuse Warning Network (DAWN), operated by the National Institute on Drug Abuse. This system uses information provided by hospitals and emergency rooms. DAWN data indicate that between 1976 and 1981 the incidence of cocaine-related medical emergencies and deaths tripled and that during 1983 there was a dramatic increase in emergency room mentions associated with cocaine. Furthermore, cocaine in combination with other drugs is cited as the cause of more than 66% of emergency room episodes involving cocaine. According to the DAWN reports, speedballing (the combination of heroin and cocaine) was the second most frequently mentioned combination. Other drugs used in combination with cocaine included tranquilizers, alcohol, and marijuana. People under 20 years of age most frequently use marijuana in combination with cocaine. Admissions to public treatment programs for cocaine-related problems have in-

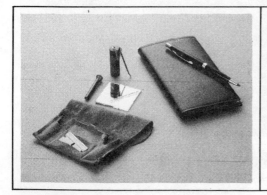

In the early 1980s cocaine abuse spread throughout middle class and business communities. The pervasiveness of the problem is demonstrated by the marketing of compact "executive kits," like the one pictured here, which contain all the items needed for inconspicuous cocaine use.

creased five-fold since 1976 and this upward trend appears to be continuing. In 1983 primary cocaine problems accounted for 7.3% of all drug clinic admissions, and in the first 6 months of 1984 this figure had risen to 13.9%.

Who Uses Cocaine?

People who use or abuse cocaine represent all racial, geographical, and occupational groups of society. A 1982 study showed that among people aged 18 to 44 the prevalence of use in males (28%) was higher than in females (16.3%), but recent surveys indicate that this gender gap is narrowing. Though the percentage is higher for whites (23.7%), use by other races is a significant 15.3%. In the United States, use is greatest in the West (34.1%), but even in the South 15.8% of adults aged 18 to 44 report having used cocaine at least once.

In the past, cocaine use was usually associated with professional people such as physicians, attorneys, star athletes, and those in the entertainment business. Its high cost made it the "champagne of drugs" and it was generally restricted to people with a considerable disposable income. Until recently, most regular cocaine users earned an average income of over $25,000 per year and many were spending over $500 a week on cocaine. In some extreme cases, individuals spent as much as $3,200 in one week to support their cocaine habit.

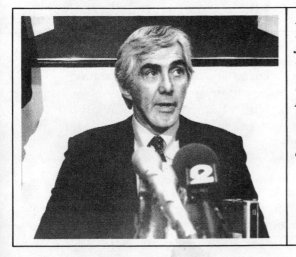

Automobile manufacturer John De Lorean was indicted in 1982 for allegedly trying to smuggle 27 kilograms of cocaine into the U.S. He was acquitted, but his case and other arrests pointed to the fact that trafficking in cocaine is not restricted to conventional criminal and counter-culture types.

Today, however, neither economic nor work status appears to be a significant barrier to use of this drug—24.3% of working adults and 15.3% of unemployed adults have used cocaine. From 1975 to the early 1980s the use of cocaine among high school seniors also increased, but this trend has leveled off. However, given the glamour associated with cocaine and the reduction of its price, many people fear that cocaine use may become even more prevalent among high school students.

Patterns of Use

Many, if not most, cocaine users take the drug for social and recreational purposes. Often it is ingested intranasally at a party where other drugs such as alcohol and marijuana are also present. It is in social contexts such as this that most people initiate cocaine use. A smaller group of users take cocaine for more specific reasons—to reduce food consumption, increase activity, decrease boredom and feelings of depression, and enhance energy and performance at work. In addition, there are other people who have been classified as intensive cocaine users. The most extreme are the compulsive users who have taken the drug frequently over a long period of time. These individuals exhibit a reduction in normal social functioning and in performance. They also tend to be preoccupied with obtaining and using cocaine.

The way cocaine is used has changed over the last 15 years. Most importantly, users have begun to experiment with new methods of use. Previously, the intranasal, and to a small extent the intravenous, route of administration was used. Around 1977 cocaine freebasing entered the scene, and an increasing number of users (approximately 5%) prefer this route. However, snorting cocaine is still by far the predominant method of administering the drug.

Of those individuals seeking treatment for cocaine problems, approximately 16% smoke cocaine, 25% inject it, and 57% snort it. Many reports indicate that smoking and taking cocaine intravenously more readily lead to compulsive cocaine use. That is not to say that snorting cocaine never results in compulsive use; it may just do so more slowly.

There is also a great deal of evidence that people who use cocaine have had previous experience with other drugs, particularly marijuana. Of those individuals who have used cocaine, 98% have also used marijuana. In addition, the frequency of marijuana use seems to be correlated with the probability of cocaine use. The greater the frequency of one's marijuana use, the more likely one is to use cocaine. This pattern is also similar among high school seniors—84% of cocaine users have also used marijuana. Furthermore, these individuals also report a significant use of alcohol and cigarettes. Data collected from the Gallup Poll indicate that alcohol, marijuana, tranquilizers, opiates, and amphetamines are the drugs most frequently used in combination with cocaine. In fact, drug use confined to a single drug is not a usual pattern for any type of drug of abuse. Most people who use psychoactive drugs take a variety of drugs, frequently in combination.

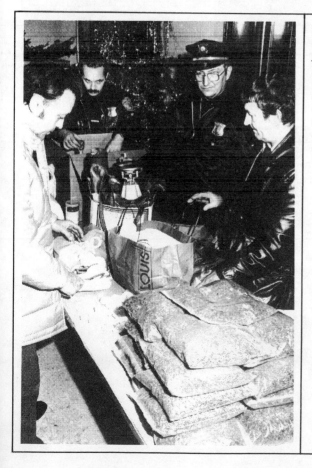

In addition to large amounts of cocaine, Boston police confiscated bags of marijuana in this 1980 drug bust. The majority of cocaine users have abused other drugs, most frequently marijuana and alcohol, and often combine the use of one with another.

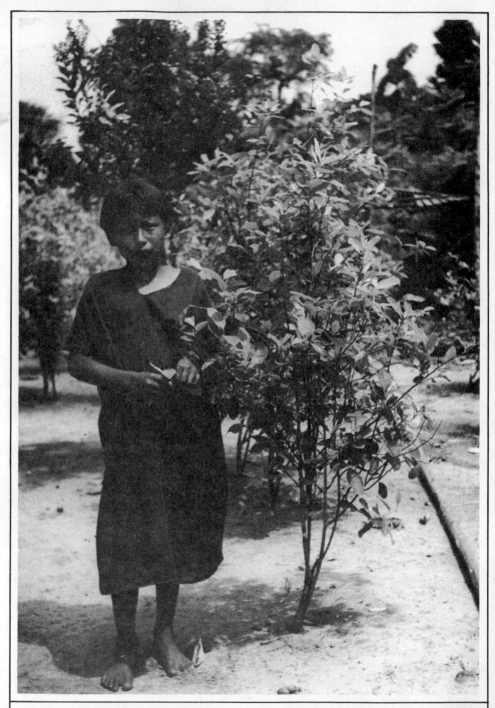

A Siona Indian boy stands beside a coca plant in Colombia. Many South American farmers depend on the coca crop as a main source of income.

CHAPTER 4

FROM THE FIELD TO THE USER

*T*he coca plant, primarily the *E. coca* species, is cultivated almost exclusively in South America, particularly in the mountain valleys of Peru, Bolivia, Colombia, Ecuador, and Brazil. Bolivian coca contains approximately 0.85% cocaine HCl (hydrochloride) as compared to Colombian coca, which contains less than 0.60% cocaine HCl. Bolivian coca is marketed as the hydrochloride powder, while the Colombian version is primarily used for the production of coca paste consumed by South Americans.

Cocaine HCl is produced in two steps. First, dried coca leaves are soaked in bicarbonate and covered with kerosene and allowed to steep. Then, varying amounts of sulfuric acid, water, and calcium carbonate are added. This process is designed to remove the cocaine alkaloids from the coca leaves. The end product is the coca paste. It takes at least 200 kg (kilograms) of leaves to produce 1 kg of paste. Next, the paste is converted to cocaine crystals, the hydrochloride. This process is relatively complicated, requiring several steps and various chemicals such as ether, alcohol, ammonia, and hydrochloric acid. Sometimes coca paste is converted to cocaine paste, which is then transported to other laboratories (usually in Colombia), where it is finally converted to the water-soluble cocaine hydrochloride. Approximately 2.5 kg of coca paste are needed to produce 1 kg of cocaine HCl, but this can vary depending on the efficiency of the process as well as the purity of the materials.

Price and Supply

There is almost no reliable way to estimate how much coca is grown and how much cocaine is produced by the South American countries. It is relatively well known that the majority of coca plants are cultivated in Peru, Bolivia, and Colombia. In addition, unknown quantities are grown in Ecuador and Brazil. As a result of more stringent trafficking

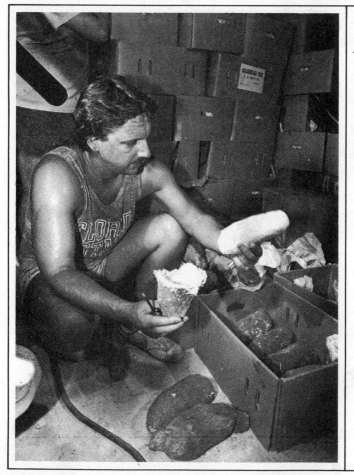

A U.S. Customs agent in Miami discovers a packet of cocaine disguised as a yam among a shipment of Colombian goods. Concealing large amounts of cocaine in cargo shipments is common practice among today's drug smugglers.

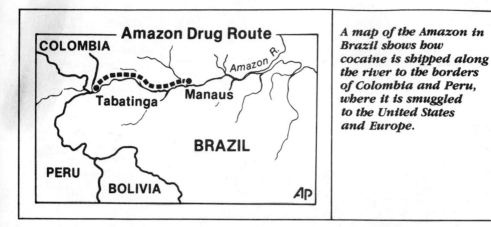

A map of the Amazon in Brazil shows how cocaine is shipped along the river to the borders of Colombia and Peru, where it is smuggled to the United States and Europe.

in Colombia, there has been an increased demand on other South American countries to expand coca cultivation. However, the extent of new production areas is still a matter of speculation.

Many believe that the rise in cocaine abuse in the last decade has been due to some extent to the reduction in its price, partially a reflection of an increase in its production and subsequent availability. In Miami in 1981, the wholesale cost of 1 kg of cocaine was $55,000. The price dropped to $25,000 in 1984, but there is now an indication that the cost is again on the rise. This may reflect the impact that increased surveillance and law enforcement measures have had on cocaine traffickers.

Despite generally decreased wholesale prices, in most American cities the cost of street cocaine has remained stable at approximately $80 to $120 per gram. In some cases the price has dropped to as low as $50 to $75 per gram, and in New York City grams selling for less than $50 have occasionally been reported. At the same time, the purity of cocaine has increased from 15%–20% to 35% or better, most likely reflecting an abundant supply.

How Cocaine Gets to the United States

The bulk of cocaine HCl is smuggled into the United States through Colombia. Much of the coca paste produced in Peru and Bolivia is first smuggled into Colombia, where it is refined and then shipped to the United States or other countries. Cocaine is probably transported from Colombia because of

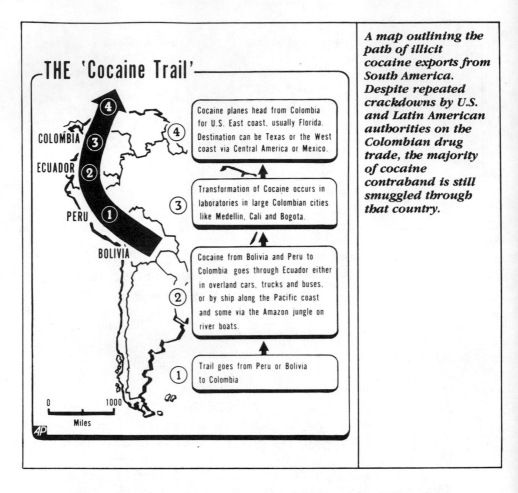

THE 'Cocaine Trail'

COLOMBIA
ECUADOR
PERU
BOLIVIA

④ Cocaine planes head from Colombia for U.S. East coast, usually Florida. Destination can be Texas or the West coast via Central America or Mexico.

③ Transformation of Cocaine occurs in laboratories in large Colombian cities like Medellin, Cali and Bogota.

② Cocaine from Bolivia and Peru to Colombia goes through Ecuador either in overland cars, trucks and buses, or by ship along the Pacific coast and some via the Amazon jungle on river boats.

① Trail goes from Peru or Bolivia to Colombia

0   1000
    Miles

A map outlining the path of illicit cocaine exports from South America. Despite repeated crackdowns by U.S. and Latin American authorities on the Colombian drug trade, the majority of cocaine contraband is still smuggled through that country.

this country's convenient geographic location. From there traffickers can easily transport the drug via ships or nonstop commercial flights—as cargo or air mail or hidden within personal belongings. One recent trend in smuggling is to conceal large quantities of cocaine in cargo shipments aboard both commercial and noncommercial seafaring vessels. The amount of drugs seized from commercial vessels grew from 93 kg in 1981 to 1,729 kg just two years later.

Because of the current overproduction of cocaine, rather than transporting the paste to Colombia, countries such as Bolivia are beginning to process it themselves and then traffic the cocaine directly to the United States. Bolivia's increased interest in the illegal cocaine trade will undoubtedly lead to strict competition with traffickers in Colombia, particularly since Colombia relies heavily on other South American countries to provide the cocaine to be smuggled.

Regardless of changes in trade patterns, a recent estimate indicates that approximately 75% of the cocaine HCl smuggled into the United States still arrives via Colombia. Bermuda and Latin America, particularly Mexico, are intermediate transport areas where small private planes can refuel. Over 60% of cocaine is transported to the United States by general aviation aircraft, which can hold as much as 1,000 kg. It is very difficult to intercept drugs smuggled by air because there are hundreds of airstrips throughout the numerous remote areas of Latin America and these aircraft can take off and land easily without detection. In addition, often the cargo is dropped far from landing strips and law enforcement agents.

Although most cocaine is destined for the United States, an increasing amount is also being smuggled into other countries such as Canada and various European nations.

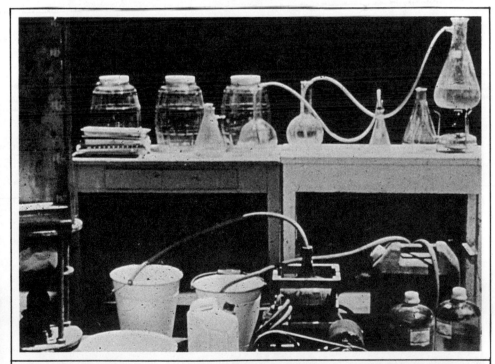

The bulk of coca leaves is transported to small cocaine labs in Colombia, where it is converted into cocaine hydrochloride. Compared with the profits, the cost of processing the leaves is minimal.

The Control of Trafficking

The United States Drug Enforcement Administration (DEA), which is responsible for the regulation of drugs, has agents throughout Latin and South America promoting antidrug activities. In the past, officials of the South American countries have done little to assist the DEA in its efforts to control the illicit drug trade. Recently there has been an increase in cooperation by the governments of Colombia and several other Latin American countries. Political pressure from the United States has been largely responsible for this change, but, in addition, Colombia is becoming increasingly aware that her own citizens are suffering from the effects of coca paste.

One method of controlling trafficking is to limit the supply of chemicals, such as ether and acetone, essential to cocaine production. In fact, since 1983 Colombia has imposed strict regulations on the importation of specific chemicals for this reason.

An increasingly popular means of controlling cocaine supply is to destroy the coca plant. However, this plant is very difficult to eradicate manually and there is considerable

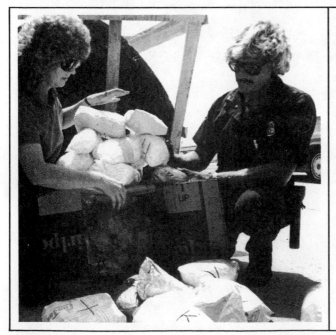

In Miami, U.S. Customs agents unload 39 kilograms of cocaine discovered in an aircraft nose cone by a drug-sniffing dog. The smugglers had unsuccessfully attempted to camouflage the drug's scent by packing it among green peppers.

controversy over using airborne pesticides. Also, for many South American farmers illicit coca production is their only source of income. Unfortunately, there are virtually no alternative crops that could bring in a fraction of the income brought in by coca production.

Regardless of the means used in attempting to decrease the cocaine supply, success will be difficult because cocaine trafficking is a big business that brings in considerable sums of money to otherwise poor countries. For instance, the Bolivian coca crop brings in nearly $2 billion a year—3 times the amount received from legal exports. To adequately control illicit coca production, distribution, and use, many factors have to be dealt with. An increase in drug abuse treatment and enforcement is crucial. Furthermore, research related to treatment and the causes of drug abuse needs to be undertaken to add to current knowledge of cocaine and its actions. Finally, international cooperation, which must include helping farmers make the transition from cocaine to other, legal crops, is essential.

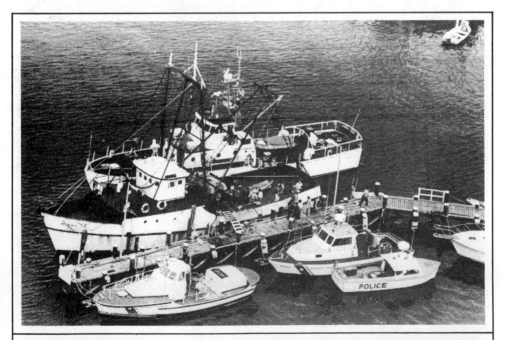

U.S. authorities seize a drug-smuggling ship. Despite strict border patrols, under 10% of the drugs coming into the U.S. are intercepted.

A graph illustrating how an intravenous injection of cocaine alters the brain activity, eye movements, and the respiratory and heart rates of a rhesus monkey. By observing the responses of different animals to cocaine, researchers hope to reach a better understanding of the drug's physical and emotional effects on human beings.

CHAPTER 5

SCIENTIFIC STUDIES OF COCAINE'S EFFECTS

Psychologists, behavioral scientists, and pharmacologists have known since the 1960s that the properties of drugs that are responsible for their abuse can be studied in the laboratory using animal subjects. Though it is well known that the physiological effects of any drug can be studied using animals, it has not always been appreciated that animals can also be used to study a drug's effects on behavior.

Over the last 20 years an animal model of drug dependence has been developed. Scientists have shown that animals such as rats and rhesus monkeys will readily learn to push a lever in order to receive an injection of the very same drugs that humans abuse. These drugs include heroin, barbiturates, and psychomotor stimulants such as amphetamine and cocaine. In contrast, drugs that are not abused by any substantial portion of the population are not self-administered voluntarily by animals. In fact, when given the opportunity, animals will actually try to escape or avoid the injection of these drugs. Like many humans, animals find them unpleasant.

It is well known that animals will learn to perform complex behaviors to obtain a reward of food or water. Behavioral scientists refer to such rewards as positive reinforcers. Experiments have shown that drugs can also act as positive reinforcers. What this means is that behavior leading to the injection of a drug will be repeated at an increased frequency as long as the behavior is rewarded with the drug. Scientists believe that the extent of a drug's reinforcing properties is related to the drug's abuse potential. The greater the drug's reinforcing properties, the greater its potential for abuse. Though there are always dangers in extrapolating from animal studies of any nature, the self-administration studies on cocaine provide good evidence that this drug has powerful reinforcing properties.

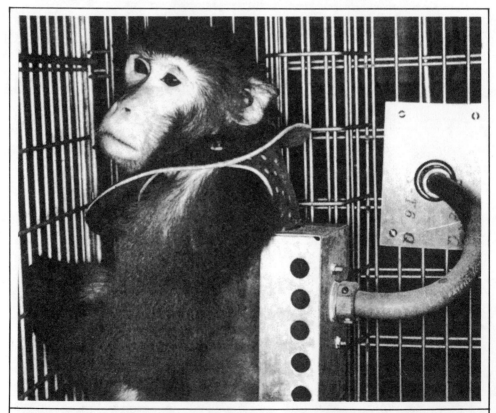

When rhesus monkeys were hooked up to a device that administers cocaine, they consistently repeated behavior that yielded a cocaine injection, even when the drug was accompanied by an electric shock.

The Self-Administration Design

Drugs are usually given to animals intravenously. With the rhesus monkey this involves surgically implanting an intravenous catheter, or small rubber tube, into a major vein. The animal is then fitted with a steel harness that is connected to the wall of its cage by a metal spring, through which the catheter runs. This arrangement allows the monkey to move relatively freely within the confines of the cage, which is equipped with response levers and lights that signal drug availability.

In most experiments, when an animal presses the lever it automatically receives a measured dose of a drug such as cocaine. What is important to remember is that animals are not coerced to make this response. Because of their natural inquisitiveness, monkeys are quick to explore their environment. This exploratory behavior ultimately leads to an accidental pushing of the lever, resulting in the delivery of the drug to the animal's bloodstream. Within hours (sometimes minutes) the animal learns the association between its lever-pushing behavior and the effects of the cocaine and begins to press the lever regularly.

Self-Administration of Cocaine

There is considerable evidence from scientific studies that cocaine is a positive reinforcer. In one study, rhesus monkeys were required to press a lever once in order to receive a single intravenous dose. There was no punishment for not pressing the lever, other than being denied cocaine. The monkeys were allowed to do this for a period of 4 hours each day, during which time they repeatedly pressed the lever and became highly intoxicated.

Cocaine is believed to be one of the most reinforcing drugs and has been self-administered by all routes by rats, dogs, squirrel and rhesus monkeys, and baboons. Furthermore, the drug can be self-administered under a variety of experimental circumstances. A researcher can alter the amount of work an animal must do before receiving the drug. For example, an animal may have to press a lever 10 times for each injection of cocaine. In some cases, the animal has to wait a specific amount of time before a specific behavior will be rewarded with cocaine. Regardless of the complexity of the behavior required of the animal, cocaine maintains high levels of behavior because of its great reinforcing property.

Reinforcing Strength

Many experimental designs have been used to measure directly the strength of a drug's reinforcing properties. One design uses the progressive ratio schedule, which gradually increases the number of times the animal has to press a lever to receive the drug. For example, the first injection may require 10 presses, the second 20, the third 40, and so forth. This continues until the breaking point is reached—the point at which the animal ceases to respond.

Using this procedure monkeys have been shown to press a lever as many as 6,400 to 12,800 times for a single injection of cocaine. The breaking point for cocaine is much higher than for other stimulant drugs such as amphetamine, suggesting that cocaine's reinforcing properties, and thus its potential for abuse, are greater.

Cocaine's reinforcing strength was also demonstrated in studies that gave rhesus monkeys the opportunity to choose between cocaine and other positive reinforcers. Data show that at most doses cocaine was preferred over procaine, a local anesthetic, and diethylpropion, a CNS stimulant. When given the choice between cocaine and the opportunity to have visual contact with other monkeys, the monkeys chose the drug. And even more startling, monkeys will choose cocaine over food even to the point of starvation.

Animals will even self-administer cocaine when each injection is accompanied by an electric shock. When given a choice between receiving a high dose of cocaine with an electric shock and receiving a low dose with no shock, animals selected the drug with the shock. Obviously, cocaine is a very potent reinforcer.

The Consequences of an Unlimited Supply

The toxic effects of cocaine have also been investigated using self-administration procedures. In most of the studies discussed above, cocaine was available only for a limited period each day. Under these conditions, though the animals became obviously intoxicated, severe drug toxicity was rare. However, when cocaine is available 24 hours per day rhesus monkeys sometimes ingest up to 100 mg per kg (kilogram) of body weight, doses high enough to produce convulsions that lead to death. Thus it seems that when drug availability is unlimited, animals, including humans, may increase their drug-taking behavior to the extent of severe toxicity and even death.

In summary, laboratory experiments have provided much data to support and predict the extent and debilitating effects of cocaine use among humans. Cocaine is a strong reinforcer under a variety of conditions. Animals, including people, will go to great lengths to get cocaine, will choose it over almost all other reinforcers including food, and will continue to take the drug even when such behavior is punished. These results help to explain the loss of control that many cocaine users exhibit.

Cocaine and the Brain

Though it is known that cocaine, one of the most powerful reinforcers, has a high abuse potential, the underlying neural mechanisms by which cocaine, as well as other drugs, exerts its rewarding properties are not clearly understood. Biological psychologists claim that psychological states such as euphoria, depression, and aggression all have an underlying physiological and neurochemical basis. Therefore, it is presumed that drugs of abuse are reinforcing because they activate reward centers in the brain. Numerous studies have attempted to locate the brain circuitry responsible for this reinforcement. In addition, research using cocaine has focused on the brain mechanisms responsible for this drug's addictive properties. Such studies also add to our knowledge concerning the reinforcing characteristics of feeding and sexual behavior.

The initial evidence suggesting the existence of a neural mechanism for reward was obtained using a technique called brain stimulation. Researchers surgically implanted electrodes in the brains of rats and through these electrodes applied electrical stimulation to very specific areas. It was found that the rats would press a lever in order to receive stimulation in certain areas of the brain but not in others. Such findings led researchers to conclude that there are areas of the brain that when stimulated induce pleasure. Further studies indicated that certain chemicals in the brain—the catecholamines norepinephrine and dopamine—were involved in these reward mechanisms. Since psychomotor stimulants such as cocaine and amphetamine are rewarding and are known to activate catecholamine systems, it is reasonable to conclude that reinforcing drugs activate the same reward circuits as electrical stimulation.

There is considerable evidence that cocaine and amphetamine exert their rewarding actions by increasing the amount of the neurotransmitters norepinephrine (NE) and dopamine (DA) present at the synapse. Both cocaine and amphetamine block the reuptake of these neurotransmitters after their release from the axon terminal and thus prevent their inactivation. In addition, amphetamine causes the release of these neurotransmitters. Drugs that interfere with the production of these substances (synthesis blockers) or block their action at the receptors (antagonists) reduce the rewarding effects of both cocaine and amphetamine. While both NE and DA may be important in mediating the rein-

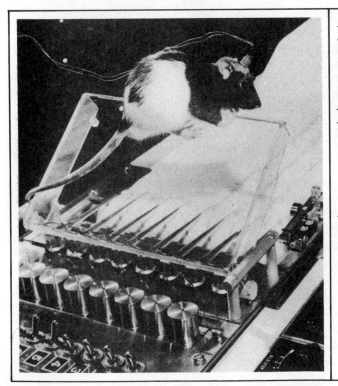

Electrodes have been surgically implanted in the heads of laboratory rats to locate specific reward centers in the brain, areas that produce sensations of pleasure when electrically excited. Stimulants such as cocaine appear to induce pleasure in the same regions of the brain that respond positively to electrical stimulation, suggesting a biochemical explanation for cocaine's appeal.

forcing actions of cocaine, recent studies indicate a greater role for DA. For instance, animals will perform to receive drugs that specifically interact with DA receptors, though this is not true for direct NE receptor activators.

Human studies confirm the animal data. Drugs that block NE and DA, or specifically DA, reduce the euphoric effects produced by intravenous amphetamine in humans. This block does not occur if a drug that only interferes with NE is given, again suggesting that DA may be the most important neurotransmitter for reinforcement. Many scientists believe that dopamine is important for mediating all kinds of reward, but this theory is still controversial.

Not only are specific chemicals in the brain involved in reward systems but there are specific brain areas as well. Anatomically, an area of the limbic system (where feelings of emotion are thought to emanate) called the nucleus accumbens appears to be important in mediating reward. Destruction of this area reduces or eliminates the reinforcing properties of both amphetamine and cocaine. Furthermore, amphetamine injected directly into this area of the brain acts as a reward to rats, whereas injections into other areas do not produce these effects.

Although studies that focus on cocaine's action on the brain are important in and of themselves, their findings have broader implications. The rewarding actions of these drugs are thought to act via the same neural circuitry as the actions of natural rewards. The cocaine-induced euphoria and elevated mood appears to be a result of the activation of neural systems that evolved to serve the control of behavior by natural reinforcers such as food and water. The most recent evidence suggests that both drugs and rewarding brain stimulation activate these natural reward systems in the brain, and by studying one kind of reward, knowledge about reward systems in general will result.

Studying cocaine's effects on the brain also increases knowledge about how the brain works. For example, understanding how cocaine produces convulsions may lead to diagnosis and treatment of epilepsy. And if, in fact, the 'toxic psychosis induced by high doses of cocaine is the result of an alteration of the same mechanisms that cause schizophrenia, knowledge of one can increase our understanding of the other.

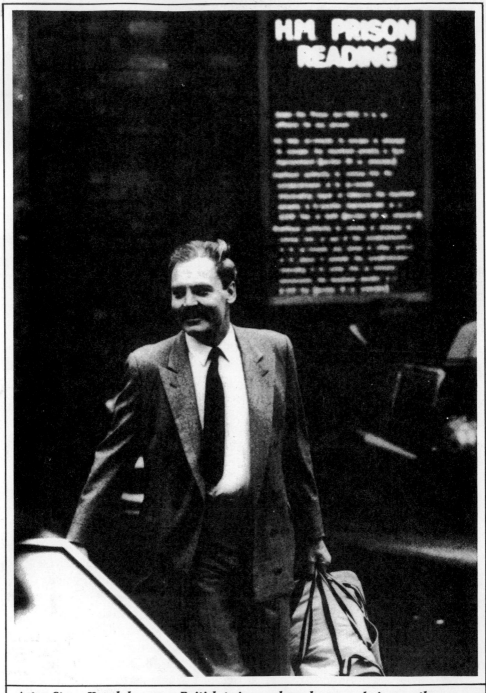

Actor Stacy Keach leaves a British prison, where he served six months for attempting to smuggle cocaine into England. Since his release Keach has lectured widely on the perils of drug abuse.

CHAPTER 6

TREATMENT FOR COCAINE ABUSE

The current epidemic of cocaine abuse has led to a tremendous increase in the need and demand for treatment. Unfortunately, this rapid rise in abuse has not been met with an adequate number of effective treatment methods. A similar situation existed during the cocaine epidemic in the 19th century. At that time many of the treatments were little better than no treatment at all. For instance, home cures, some of which even contained cocaine as well as other drugs of abuse such as alcohol and morphine, were used to help patients withdraw from cocaine. The danger, of course, was that these drugs also had high abuse potentials. Sometimes cocaine abusers were treated using hypnosis or sent to sanitariums, where treatment included living in a drug-free environment, receiving moral lectures, eating healthy foods, and exercising regularly. Upon their release, patients often relapsed immediately. In effect, there were no successful treatments for cocaine abuse until well into the 20th century. Though the situation is not much better today, there are types of therapy that have proven moderately successful.

Choosing the Best Treatment

Before deciding on a particular form of treatment it is important that the specific needs of the patient are carefully evaluated. There are three essential considerations. The first is the severity of the problem, which can vary significantly.

The amount and regularity of cocaine used and its route of administration are important factors in determining the seriousness of the drug problem. In general, the risk of suffering from harmful effects increases with length of use and when cocaine is taken intravenously or by freebasing. On the other hand, serious problems can arise in users who have only been taking cocaine intranasally and only for a short time. Regardless, the choice of treatment must in part be based upon the severity of the problem. For instance, some patients realize early on that they are having trouble controlling their cocaine use. Others do not seek treatment until they have lost nearly everything—money, spouses, friends, and jobs. Clearly, for these people simply stopping cocaine use will not be a plausible method of treatment since they have so little left in their lives that can compete with the cocaine. Suffice it to say, the earlier the patient seeks help, the easier and more successful the treatment will be.

The second consideration in choosing a proper form of treatment of cocaine abuse involves establishing whether or

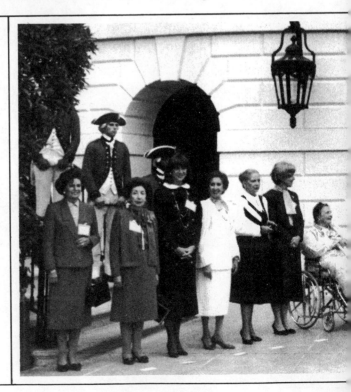

First Lady Nancy Reagan meets with 17 first ladies of other nations who attended a two-day conference in Washington on drugs. Mrs. Reagan has waged a highly publicized anti-drug-abuse campaign that has been targeted especially to young people; however, the Reagan administration's budget for drug education programs dropped from $14 million in 1981 to under $3 million in 1985.

not there are accompanying psychological disorders. Cocaine users may be suffering from an underlying depression or attention disorder and using cocaine as a form of self-medication. Just stopping the cocaine abuse will not cure the other deep-seated problems. In fact, in some cases it may actually make them worse, at least for a short time. Therefore an effective treatment program must include ways of dealing with both the psychological *and* the cocaine problems. There has been an ongoing debate in the medical field about whether the psychological problems lead to cocaine abuse or are the result of the cocaine intoxication. But on a practical level this distinction may be academic since both the drug abuse problem and the psychological disorders must be treated.

The third consideration in selecting a mode of treatment involves complications from excessive cocaine use that must be treated immediately. Patients who have taken a great deal of cocaine in the recent past may be in a state of agitation or may have even become psychotic. In both cases, their

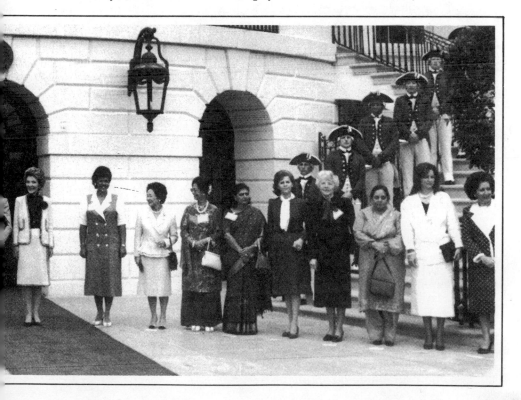

well-being is in jeopardy and immediate measures must be taken. Agitation, which in severe cases can include convulsive-like symptoms, is often treated with Valium or some other kind of sedative/hypnotic. Psychotic symptoms, which can include hallucinations and delirium, are usually treated with neuroleptics, antipsychotic tranquilizers such as Thorazine. However, such treatment can be risky. There is some evidence that such medication can precipitate convulsions in patients with cocaine-induced psychosis.

Some patients seek treatment following a binge with cocaine. They often experience an extreme form of crashing that makes their symptoms indistinguishable from those of severe depression. Since these patients are often in danger of committing suicide, it is important that they be kept under close observation within a hospital setting. Allowing such patients to catch up on their sleep, which the cocaine run has disrupted, and providing a controlled environment is a first step. Only then, however, can treatment for the abuse problem itself be considered. In addition to psychological complications there is also the possibility of the physical complications previously discussed. These problems, particularly when life threatening, must be dealt with before treatment for actual cocaine abuse begins. In some cases, such medical problems may persist even while the patient is receiving therapy for his or her cocaine problem.

Treatment for cocaine abuse must be based upon an assessment of each individual that takes into consideration the severity of the abuse problem, the possibility of underlying psychological problems, and the existence of acute psychiatric or medical complications. If success is to be expected, the treatment must carefully fit all the needs of each patient.

Conventional Treatments

All the formal types of therapy utilized today are psychological and do not involve the use of drugs. Many have been adapted from treatments used for other types of drug abuse, and in all cases their effectiveness has not been absolutely proven. These therapies will be described here separately, though in most settings they are used in combinations. And again, it is important to consider the individual patient's needs when designing a treatment program.

Initially, one must decide if it is necessary to begin treatment within a hospital setting. For some individuals, such as those with severe depression or intense craving for the drug, it may be essential. For others, it may be a matter of choice. An advantage of a hospital is that the therapist has greater control and can provide almost constant treatment. On the other hand, as the sanitarium experience of the 19th century showed, the problem of cocaine abuse needs to be dealt with in the patient's normal day-to-day setting. As with prisoners, merely removing people from the situation may not allow them to learn to control their own behaviors.

Contingency Contracting

One of the most controversial forms of behavioral treatment uses contracts that specify a negative consequence for patients who are not complying with their prescribed treatment. These consequences can be extremely harsh and even include the loss of a job or a huge financial penalty. A relapse can be detected by monitoring a patient's urine. If it is found to contain cocaine, or if the patient refuses to furnish the urine, the agreed upon consequences will be invoked by the therapist. For instance, many patients write letters to their employers, parents, or, in the case of some professionals, their

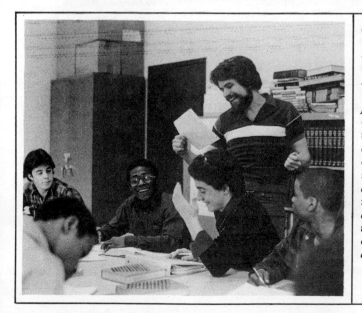

Supportive therapies have achieved some success in treating cocaine abusers. The Phoenix House drug rehabilitation center provides educational workshops and a drug-free environment where, under the care of qualified counselors, recovering drug abusers can share with each other their experiences, feelings, and problems.

licensing board, stating that they have a cocaine problem. These letters are held by the therapist and are not sent unless the patient fails the contract. As long as the patient remains off cocaine, the therapist keeps the letters. This form of therapy has proven very successful, but usually only for as long as the contract is in effect.

Many people have criticized this treatment, claiming that it is unethical because a single relapse results in severe punishment. Also, it can be argued that in the beginning of treatment many patients feel desperate and may be willing to agree to anything just to prove to themselves and others that they are doing something about their problem. It should be remembered, however, that the consequences have been agreed to by the patient with the full realization that a harsh punishment will accompany failure. The general technique appears to have value. If it is modified to include more positive and less severe consequences and if the contents of the contract are continually reviewed, the acceptability of this approach may increase.

Desensitization

Another form of treatment used for many types of excessive behavior and phobia problems is known as systematic desensitization. It is based upon the idea that certain kinds of

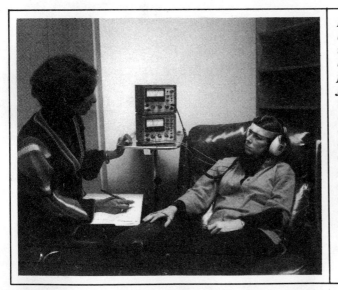

Proponents of biofeedback therapy maintain that one can learn to control physiological functions formerly thought to be involuntary. By using biofeedback equipment, recovering cocaine abusers can develop relaxation techniques that may alleviate the anxiety and psychological craving that accompany cocaine withdrawal.

situations in a person's environment arouse anxiety or, in the case of the cocaine, craving that triggers the use of drugs. Proponents of this treatment method contend that patients can learn to face these situations without resorting to drugs. In this learning process the patient first thinks of those objects and/or situations that would normally lead to anxiety or craving. Then, with the help of the therapist, the patient orders these stimuli according to the intensity of their effects, usually in increasing order. The therapist then presents these stimuli, either verbally and/or with visual aids, and teaches the patient to relax despite their presence. The therapist starts with the least threatening stimulus and moves up the hierarchy. The relaxation exercises usually consist of muscle relaxation training but can also utilize biofeedback techniques and even hydrotherapy (relaxing while immersed in water) and massage. Though this approach has been successful in treating some phobias, its usefulness in helping cocaine abusers remains unproven.

Assertiveness Training

Another therapy approach, assertiveness training, is based on the assumption that for a variety of reasons some people are simply unable to say no. Applied to drug use, assertiveness training begins with the understanding that the cocaine abuser is constantly under pressure from drug dealers and fellow drug users to continue cocaine use. The treatment consists of having the patient practice refusing cocaine in various simulated situations in which use of the drug might be particularly tempting. Even though the simplicity of this approach is appealing, its effectiveness has not been evaluated.

Supportive Therapies

In addition to behavioral treatments, supportive therapies or more classical psychotherapies have also been used to treat cocaine abusers. These approaches involve helping patients disentangle themselves from lifestyles that revolve around cocaine use. They are encouraged to avoid friends and social situations that involve cocaine. Therapy can also include educating patients about the actions and dangers of cocaine and helping them overcome the difficulties that have resulted from excessive cocaine abuse.

As previously mentioned, many people who are cocaine abusers have other psychological problems that require treatment. In many cases these problems predate the person's cocaine use, and thus there is little reason to believe that the problems will suddenly disappear when cocaine use stops. Unless these problems are alleviated the discontinuation of cocaine use can be almost impossible. But again, the exact nature of the supportive therapy or psychotherapy required depends to a great extent on the individual needs of the patient.

Self-Help Treatments

There has recently been an explosion of self-help techniques designed to assist the cocaine abuser in treating himself or herself. How useful they are, however, is totally unknown at this time. Some techniques even include suggestions as to how to continue to use cocaine safely, a highly questionable approach. Books describing these techniques often include educational materials as well as suggestions about alternative

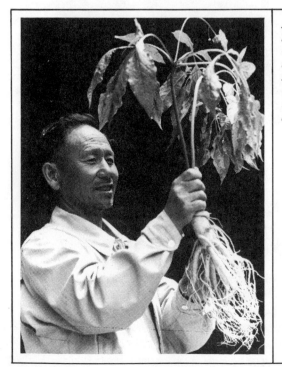

A Korean farmer displays a harvested ginseng plant. Concoctions made from ginseng are among the mildly stimulating herbal remedies that have been proposed for use as aids in overcoming the cocaine habit.

activities such as running. Though many of the self-help ideas set forth in these books may be valuable and, in fact, very similar to those used in formal treatment therapies, in most cases their usefulness outside a therapeutic environment has not been scientifically proven.

Some self-help manuals suggest diets that supposedly will allow one to stop cocaine use. Others include treatments designed to help the user alleviate the problems associated with withdrawal and to reverse some of the damaging health effects resulting from excessive cocaine use. For example, some people believe that the depletion of certain chemicals in the brain, such as catecholamines, is responsible for the crashing during withdrawal and the continued feelings of craving. Supposedly, taking amino acid supplements and hormone precursors (substances from which hormones are formed), such as tyrosine, along with maintaining adequate nutrition can reverse these effects. Drugs such as l-tryptophan are often promoted to help cocaine users sleep adequately during the initial withdrawal phase. Some believe that vitamin insufficiency and dehydration can be alleviated by ingesting electrolyte fluids with glucose and vitamin C. It has also been suggested that, since the stimulant cocaine is so dangerous, users should switch to other types of stimulants such as over-the-counter preparations containing phenylpropanolamine. Herbal remedies containing such compounds as ginseng have also become part of this self-cure approach. Even coca leaves have been suggested as a therapeutic alternative.

Even though many of these suggestions may be useful or, at the very least, not harmful, it must be emphasized that it is most difficult for a person to stop cocaine abuse without outside help. Fortunately, some of these self-help books also include a list of treatment facilities and referrals for those who come to realize that their problem requires more formal treatment.

Pharmacological Treatments

The use of drugs to treat cocaine abuse is still at an experimental stage, but there are many reasons to believe that certain chemicals can be helpful. Because some people abuse cocaine in response to an underlying pathology such as depression, the pharmacological treatment could be designed with the assumption that once the psychological problem is cured the craving for cocaine will cease. Other treatments are based upon the assumption that if the effects of cocaine, such as the rush or euphoria, can be blocked by chemical means, the abuser will no longer want to continue to take cocaine. The most accepted rationale for using a chemical treatment is that chronic cocaine use has produced a neurophysiologic change in the brain, reflected in changes in behavior. Although physiological treatment aimed directly at changing that behavior is useful, greater success may be possible if drugs are given that either temporarily or permanently reverse the changes in the functioning of the brain.

Antidepressant Therapy

One type of chemical treatment uses tricyclic antidepressants, drugs used in the treatment of depression. Repeated use of cocaine produces changes in the levels of certain chemicals in the brain and changes in neural receptors that react to these same chemicals. These changes, presumed to be related to the negative feelings associated with abstinence and subsequent craving, can be reversed by tricyclic antidepressants. In addition to reversing the neurochemical changes that have been produced by cocaine, tricyclics may also be useful in actually blocking the cocaine's euphoric effects. Finally, the usefulness of tricyclics may be due to the fact that, in addition to a cocaine problem, the patient has an underlying depression, which responds to this antidepressant.

Regardless of the reason for their therapeutic action, antidepressants have been shown to be moderately successful in experimental evaluations. However, the evidence is still very minimal and far more research is required before antidepressant therapy can be considered anything but experimental.

Lithium Therapy

Lithium, normally used in the treatment of manic-depressive disorders, has also been used experimentally in the treatment of cocaine abuse. In animal studies this drug has been shown to block many of the behavioral and neurochemical effects of stimulants such as amphetamine and cocaine. Although experimental results have been variable, lithium may also be able to block the euphoria produced by these two drugs. Test results have not always been consistent, but many findings do indicate that lithium could be useful in treating cocaine abuse.

If patients ingesting lithium do not experience the sought-after euphoria, they might cease taking the drug. Of course, they might also cease taking lithium. Unfortunately, the few studies that have been done have shown variable results, and it now seems that lithium is most successful in treating cocaine abusers with certain underlying mental disorders normally treated with lithium. Whether or not this drug will prove generally useful for a large body of cocaine abusers remains to be seen.

Treatment with Other Stimulants

It has been suggested that cocaine users might be effectively treated with other, less dangerous stimulants. One such stimulant is methylphenidate (Ritalin), a drug often used in the treatment of attention disorders (hyperactivity and minimal brain syndrome) in children. There are two theoretical reasons for using this drug in the treatment of cocaine abuse.

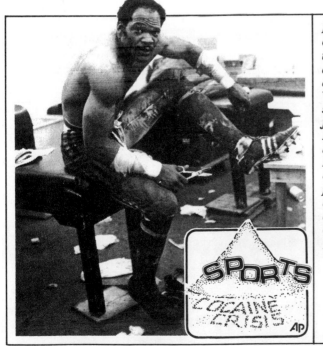

Former football player Carl Eller, who admitted to having had a serious drug problem during his days with the Minnesota Vikings, now works as a special drug consultant for the National Football League on matters of alcohol and drug abuse. In recent years, instances of cocaine abuse among professional athletes have attracted an increasing amount of media coverage and public concern.

Firstly, methylphenidate will produce a cross-tolerance to cocaine, such that methylphenidate's presence in the blood decreases or eliminates the body's sensitivity to cocaine's euphoric effects. In fact, it is methadone's cross-tolerance to heroin that makes it useful in treating heroin addiction. Even though many people do not understand the value of simply replacing one drug for another (both methylphenidate and methadone are abused), the replacement drug has the advantage of dosage control and decreased legal risk. Since the patient is getting the drug from a physician, ties with dealers and cocaine associates are broken. Though methylphenidate may be successful in treating cocaine abuse because of its cross-tolerance effects, the evidence to support its use is minimal.

Secondly, the use of methylphenidate in the treatment of cocaine abuse might be recommended if the drug abuser is actually suffering from minimal brain dysfunction (MBD), for which methylphenidate is prescribed. Because of the similarity in effects of this drug and cocaine, users of cocaine are actually engaging in self-medication.

However, many of methylphenidate's effects are similar to those of cocaine and amphetamine. This drug is addictive and at normal doses can produce side effects such as mood changes, nervousness, insomnia, dizziness, headache, appetite loss, and rapid and irregular heartbeat. Symptoms of overdose include fever, convulsions, hallucinations, and coma.

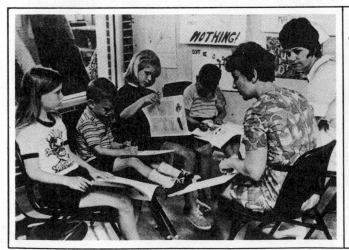

By acquainting young people with the dangers of cocaine, educators hope to reverse the tide of cocaine abuse among teenagers. The severity of the problem is illustrated by a survey which indicated that 16% of U.S. high school seniors tried cocaine in 1985.

Other Treatments

The widespread use and abuse of cocaine and its resultant problems have led to an almost frantic search for quick and easy solutions. In South America the excessive smoking of coca paste has been particularly devastating. In Peru the situation appeared so dire that a drastic form of treatment was suggested and tried. In that country, physicians have been performing a type of psychosurgery on patients who have an extensive and debilitating history of coca paste smoking. The scientific basis for this form of treatment is nonexistent, and it is likely that its use is an indication of how desperate therapists and families of cocaine abusers have become. Although this treatment, which leaves the patient profoundly changed intellectually, continues to be used in Peru, relapse to cocaine use is the rule, not the exception.

Although the need for better treatments for cocaine abuse is great, it may take a long time before a real cure is found. Even then it is unlikely that a single approach will be successful for all drug users seeking treatment. As previously emphasized, people differ in the seriousness of their cocaine use and have different needs that warrant individualized treatment. Even if successful treatments are found, the economic cost will be high. Though counseling is extremely important, it is clear that the best approach to curbing cocaine abuse is through education and prevention.

COCA-BOLA is a masticating or chewing paste made from the leaves of the Peruvian Cocoa plant. A small portion chewed occasionally acts as a powerful tonic to the muscular and nervous system, relieving fatigue and exhaustion, and enabling the user to perform additional mental and physical labor without evil after-effects.

As a remedy and substitute for TOBACCO, ALCOHOL and OPIUM, in the treatment of those habits, it is invaluable.

PROF. WM. F. WAUGH, M. D., in a paper read before the Pa. State Medical Society (*Phila. Medical Times,* March 1888), calls attention to its value for this purpose. It relieves the insufferable craving for stimulants, and prevents depression, nausea and loss of appetite, and acts as a general tonic, stimulant and sustaining agent. In this last respect it is vastly superior to all tobacco substitutes, etc., which are usually combinations of licorice root and other inert ingredients. It is harmless in its action, creates no habit, and its use can at any time be suspended.

COCOA-BOLA is put up in handsome tin pocket boxes containing sufficient for at least two weeks' use.

PRICE PER BOX, 50 CTS; BY MAIL 55 CTS.

25C mailed direct to me will bring a **Special Sample Box** with Booklet, "Coca-Bola and its Uses" Interesting and instructive

A late-19th-century advertisement recommending Coca-Bola, a cocaine-containing chewing paste, for the treatment of tobacco, alcohol, and opium addictions. Despite the manufacturer's assurance that the product was not harmful or habit-forming, many users found the reverse to be true.

APPENDIX

STATE AGENCIES
FOR THE PREVENTION AND TREATMENT
OF DRUG ABUSE

ALABAMA
Department of Mental Health
Division of Mental Illness and
  Substance Abuse Community
  Programs
200 Interstate Park Drive
P.O. Box 3710
Montgomery, AL 36193
(205) 271-9253

ALASKA
Department of Health and Social
  Services
Office of Alcoholism and Drug
  Abuse
Pouch H-05-F
Juneau, AK 99811
(907) 586-6201

ARIZONA
Department of Health Services
Division of Behavioral Health
  Services
Bureau of Community Services
Alcohol Abuse and Alcoholism
  Section
2500 East Van Buren
Phoenix, AZ 85008
(602) 255-1238

Department of Health Services
Division of Behavioral Health
  Services
Bureau of Community Services
Drug Abuse Section
2500 East Van Buren
Phoenix, AZ 85008
(602) 255-1240

ARKANSAS
Department of Human Services
Office on Alcohol and Drug Abuse
  Prevention
1515 West 7th Avenue
Suite 310
Little Rock, AR 72202
(501) 371-2603

CALIFORNIA
Department of Alcohol and Drug
  Abuse
111 Capitol Mall
Sacramento, CA 95814
(916) 445-1940

COLORADO
Department of Health
Alcohol and Drug Abuse Division
4210 East 11th Avenue
Denver, CO 80220
(303) 320-6137

CONNECTICUT
Alcohol and Drug Abuse
  Commission
999 Asylum Avenue
3rd Floor
Hartford, CT 06105
(203) 566-4145

DELAWARE
Division of Mental Health
Bureau of Alcoholism and Drug
  Abuse
1901 North Dupont Highway
Newcastle, DE 19720
(302) 421-6101

DISTRICT OF COLUMBIA
Department of Human Services
Office of Health Planning and
  Development
601 Indiana Avenue, NW
Suite 500
Washington, D.C. 20004
(202) 724-5641

FLORIDA
Department of Health and
  Rehabilitative Services
Alcoholic Rehabilitation Program
1317 Winewood Boulevard
Room 187A
Tallahassee, FL 32301
(904) 488-0396

Department of Health and
  Rehabilitative Services
Drug Abuse Program
1317 Winewood Boulevard
Building 6, Room 155
Tallahassee, FL 32301
(904) 488-0900

GEORGIA
Department of Human Resources
Division of Mental Health and
  Mental Retardation
Alcohol and Drug Section
618 Ponce De Leon Avenue, NE
Atlanta, GA 30365-2101
(404) 894-4785

HAWAII
Department of Health
Mental Health Division
Alcohol and Drug Abuse Branch
1250 Punch Bowl Street
P.O. Box 3378
Honolulu, HI 96801
(808) 548-4280

IDAHO
Department of Health and Welfare
Bureau of Preventive Medicine
Substance Abuse Section
450 West State
Boise, ID 83720
(208) 334-4368

ILLINOIS
Department of Mental Health and
  Developmental Disabilities
Division of Alcoholism
160 North La Salle Street
Room 1500
Chicago, IL 60601
(312) 793-2907

Illinois Dangerous Drugs
  Commission
300 North State Street
Suite 1500
Chicago, IL 60610
(312) 822-9860

INDIANA
Department of Mental Health
Division of Addiction Services
429 North Pennsylvania Street
Indianapolis, IN 46204
(317) 232-7816

IOWA
Department of Substance Abuse
505 5th Avenue
Insurance Exchange Building
Suite 202
Des Moines, IA 50319
(515) 281-3641

KANSAS
Department of Social Rehabilitation
Alcohol and Drug Abuse Services
2700 West 6th Street
Biddle Building
Topeka, KS 66606
(913) 296-3925

KENTUCKY
Cabinet for Human Resources
Department of Health Services
Substance Abuse Branch
275 East Main Street
Frankfort, KY 40601
(502) 564-2880

LOUISIANA
Department of Health and Human
  Resources
Office of Mental Health and
  Substance Abuse
655 North 5th Street
P.O. Box 4049
Baton Rouge, LA 70821
(504) 342-2565

MAINE
Department of Human Services
Office of Alcoholism and Drug
  Abuse Prevention
Bureau of Rehabilitation
32 Winthrop Street
Augusta, ME 04330
(207) 289-2781

MARYLAND
Alcoholism Control Administration
201 West Preston Street
Fourth Floor
Baltimore, MD 21201
(301) 383-2977

State Health Department
Drug Abuse Administration
201 West Preston Street
Baltimore, MD 21201
(301) 383-3312

MASSACHUSETTS
Department of Public Health
Division of Alcoholism
755 Boylston Street
Sixth Floor
Boston, MA 02116
(617) 727-1960

Department of Public Health
Division of Drug Rehabilitation
600 Washington Street
Boston, MA 02114
(617) 727-8617

MICHIGAN
Department of Public Health
Office of Substance Abuse Services
3500 North Logan Street
P.O. Box 30035
Lansing, MI 48909
(517) 373-8603

MINNESOTA
Department of Public Welfare
Chemical Dependency Program
  Division
Centennial Building
658 Cedar Street
4th Floor
Saint Paul, MN 55155
(612) 296-4614

MISSISSIPPI
Department of Mental Health
Division of Alcohol and Drug Abuse
1102 Robert E. Lee Building
Jackson, MS 39201
(601) 359-1297

MISSOURI
Department of Mental Health
Division of Alcoholism and Drug
  Abuse
2002 Missouri Boulevard
P.O. Box 687
Jefferson City, MO 65102
(314) 751-4942

MONTANA
Department of Institutions
Alcohol and Drug Abuse Division
1539 11th Avenue
Helena, MT 59620
(406) 449-2827

NEBRASKA
Department of Public Institutions
Division of Alcoholism and Drug Abuse
801 West Van Dorn Street
P.O. Box 94728
Lincoln, NB 68509
(402) 471-2851, Ext. 415

NEVADA
Department of Human Resources
Bureau of Alcohol and Drug Abuse
505 East King Street
Carson City, NV 89710
(702) 885-4790

NEW HAMPSHIRE
Department of Health and Welfare
Office of Alcohol and Drug Abuse
    Prevention
Hazen Drive
Health and Welfare Building
Concord, NH 03301
(603) 271-4627

NEW JERSEY
Department of Health
Division of Alcoholism
129 East Hanover Street CN 362
Trenton, NJ 08625
(609) 292-8949

Department of Health
Division of Narcotic and Drug Abuse
    Control
129 East Hanover Street CN 362
Trenton, NJ 08625
(609) 292-8949

NEW MEXICO
Health and Environment Department
Behavioral Services Division
Substance Abuse Bureau
725 Saint Michaels Drive
P.O. Box 968
Santa Fe, NM 87503
(505) 984-0020, Ext. 304

NEW YORK
Division of Alcoholism and Alcohol
    Abuse
194 Washington Avenue
Albany, NY 12210
(518) 474-5417

Division of Substance Abuse
    Services
Executive Park South
Box 8200
Albany, NY 12203
(518) 457-7629

NORTH CAROLINA
Department of Human Resources
Division of Mental Health, Mental
    Retardation and Substance Abuse
    Services
Alcohol and Drug Abuse Services
325 North Salisbury Street
Albemarle Building
Raleigh, NC 27611
(919) 733-4670

NORTH DAKOTA
Department of Human Services
Division of Alcoholism and Drug
    Abuse
State Capitol Building
Bismarck, ND 58505
(701) 224-2767

OHIO
Department of Health
Division of Alcoholism
246 North High Street
P.O. Box 118
Columbus, OH 43216
(614) 466-3543

Department of Mental Health
Bureau of Drug Abuse
65 South Front Street
Columbus, OH 43215
(614) 466-9023

OKLAHOMA
Department of Mental Health
Alcohol and Drug Programs
4545 North Lincoln Boulevard
Suite 100 East Terrace
P.O. Box 53277
Oklahoma City, OK 73152
(405) 521-0044

OREGON
Department of Human Resources
Mental Health Division
Office of Programs for Alcohol and
  Drug Problems
2575 Bittern Street, NE
Salem, OR 97310
(503) 378-2163

PENNSYLVANIA
Department of Health
Office of Drug and Alcohol
  Programs
Commonwealth and Forster Avenues
Health and Welfare Building
P.O. Box 90
Harrisburg, PA 17108
(717) 787-9857

RHODE ISLAND
Department of Mental Health,
  Mental Retardation and Hospitals
Division of Substance Abuse
Substance Abuse Administration
  Building
Cranston, RI 02920
(401) 464-2091

SOUTH CAROLINA
Commission on Alcohol and Drug
  Abuse
3700 Forest Drive
Columbia, SC 29204
(803) 758-2521

SOUTH DAKOTA
Department of Health
Division of Alcohol and Drug Abuse
523 East Capitol, Joe Foss Building
Pierre, SD 57501
(605) 773-4806

TENNESSEE
Department of Mental Health and
  Mental Retardation
Alcohol and Drug Abuse Services
505 Deaderick Street
James K. Polk Building, Fourth Floor
Nashville, TN 37219
(615) 741-1921

TEXAS
Commission on Alcoholism
809 Sam Houston State Office Building
Austin, TX 78701
(512) 475-2577

Department of Community Affairs
Drug Abuse Prevention Division
2015 South Interstate Highway 35
P.O. Box 13166
Austin, TX 78711
(512) 443-4100

UTAH
Department of Social Services
Division of Alcoholism and Drugs
150 West North Temple
Suite 350
P.O. Box 2500
Salt Lake City, UT 84110
(801) 533-6532

VERMONT
Agency of Human Services
Department of Social and
  Rehabilitation Services
Alcohol and Drug Abuse Division
103 South Main Street
Waterbury, VT 05676
(802) 241-2170

VIRGINIA
Department of Mental Health and
    Mental Retardation
Division of Substance Abuse
109 Governor Street
P.O. Box 1797
Richmond, VA 23214
(804) 786-5313

WASHINGTON
Department of Social and Health
    Service
Bureau of Alcohol and Substance
    Abuse
Office Building—44 W
Olympia, WA 98504
(206) 753-5866

WEST VIRGINIA
Department of Health
Office of Behavioral Health Services
Division on Alcoholism and Drug
    Abuse
1800 Washington Street East
Building 3 Room 451
Charleston, WV 25305
(304) 348-2276

WISCONSIN
Department of Health and Social
    Services
Division of Community Services
Bureau of Community Programs
Alcohol and Other Drug Abuse
    Program Office
1 West Wilson Street
P.O. Box 7851
Madison, WI 53707
(608) 266-2717

WYOMING
Alcohol and Drug Abuse Programs
Hathaway Building
Cheyenne, WY 82002
(307) 777-7115, Ext. 7118

GUAM
Mental Health & Substance Abuse
    Agency
P.O. Box 20999
Guam 96921

PUERTO RICO
Department of Addiction Control
    Services
Alcohol Abuse Programs
P.O. Box B-Y Rio Piedras Station
Rio Piedras, PR 00928
(809) 763-5014

Department of Addiction Control
    Services
Drug Abuse Programs
P.O. Box B-Y Rio Piedras Station
Rio Piedras, PR 00928
(809) 764-8140

VIRGIN ISLANDS
Division of Mental Health,
    Alcoholism & Drug Dependency
    Services
P.O. Box 7329
Saint Thomas, Virgin Islands 00801
(809) 774-7265

AMERICAN SAMOA
LBJ Tropical Medical Center
Department of Mental Health Clinic
Pago Pago, American Samoa 96799

TRUST TERRITORIES
Director of Health Services
Office of the High Commissioner
Saipan, Trust Territories 96950

Further Reading

Byck, Robert, ed. *Cocaine Papers: Sigmund Freud*. New York: Stonehill Publishing, 1974.

Cohen, Sidney. *Cocaine Today*. Rockville, Maryland: American Council for Drug Education, 1981.

Cohen, Sidney. *Cocaine: The Bottom Line*. Rockville, Maryland: American Council for Drug Education, 1985.

Gold, Mark S. *800–COCAINE*. New York: Bantam, 1984.

Grabowski, John. *Cocaine: Pharmacology, Effects and Treatment of Abuse*. NIDA Research Monograph, no. 50. Rockville, Maryland: U.S. Government Printing Office, 1984.

Peterson, Robert C. et al. *Cocaine: A Second Look*. Rockville, Maryland: American Council for Drug Education, 1983.

Glossary

addiction   a condition caused by repeated drug use, characterized by a compulsive urge to continue using the drug, a tendency to increase the dosage, and physiological and/or psychological dependence

alkaloid   any of various basic and bitter organic compounds found in seed plants

amphetamine   a drug that stimulates the nervous system and increases heart rate, blood pressure, and muscle tension; generally prescribed as a mood elevator, energizer, antidepressant, and appetite depressant, chronic use may cause delusions, hallucinations, paranoia, and psychosis

assertiveness training   a type of behavior therapy that seeks to bring about changes in emotional and other behavioral patterns including drug abuse by teaching the patient to assert him- or herself; with regard to drug use, this means gaining the ability to refuse a drug

attention disorder deficit (adult)   a disorder, often affecting adults who as children experienced attention disorders with hyperactivity, characterized by inattention and impulsivity, which interferes with social and occupational behavior

autonomic nervous system   the part of the peripheral nervous system, divided into the sympathetic and the parasympathetic nervous system, that controls the activity of the internal organs, including heart rate, blood pressure, respiration, and body temperature

axon   the part of the neuron along which the nerve impulse travels away from the cell body

barbiturate   a drug that causes depression of the central nervous system; generally used to reduce anxiety or to induce euphoria

biofeedback training   a training program designed to develop an individual's ability to control the autonomic, or involuntary, nervous system, and thus allow him or her to relax and even expand consciousness and self-awareness

cardiovascular   of, relating to, or involving the heart and blood vessels

catecholamines neurotransmitters, such as dopamine, epinephrine (adrenaline), and norepinephrine

central nervous system all the neural and supportive tissue inside the brain and spinal cord

cocaine the primary psychoactive ingredient in the coca plant and a behavioral stimulant

contingency contracting a form of behavioral treatment that uses contracts that specify a negative consequence for a patient who does not comply with the agreed upon treatment

cross-tolerance a condition of tolerance to one or more drugs caused by the body's tolerance to another drug

dendrite the hairlike structure which protrudes from the neural cell body and on which receptor sites are located

depression a sometimes overwhelming emotional state characterized by feelings of inadequacy and hopelessness and accompanied by a decrease in physical and psychological activity

dopamine a neurotransmitter found mainly in brain structures that play an important role in muscle control

electroencephalogram EEG; a record of the neural activity of the brain transmitted by electrodes fixed to the scalp

epilepsy any of various disorders marked by disturbed electrical rhythms of the central nervous system and typically manifested by convulsive attacks

epinephrine a neurotransmitter and hormone that is a potent stimulator of the sympathetic nervous system, producing increases in blood pressure and heart rate

freebase the cocaine alkaloid, or base, which results when the hydrochloride is removed from cocaine hydrochloride; freebasing refers to the process by which the hydrochloride is freed

hallucination a sensory impression that has no basis in external stimulation

heroin a semisynthetic opiate produced by a chemical modification of morphine

hypertension abnormally high blood pressure

intranasal route a route of drug administration by which the substance, often in powder form, is inhaled through the nasal passages

intravenous route a route of drug administration by which the substance, in liquid form, is injected into a vein

kindling   an enhanced behavioral and electrophysiological response to low levels of repeated electrical stimulation of the brain

lithium   an alkali metal effective in the treatment of mania and depression and currently used experimentally to treat cocaine abuse

local anesthetic   a substance that produces a loss of sensation, including pain, in a localized area without interaction with the central nervous system

marijuana   the leaves, flowers, buds, and/or branches of the hemp plant *Cannabis sativa* or *Cannabis indica* that contain cannabinoids, a group of intoxicating drugs

methylphenidate   Ritalin; a central nervous system stimulant chemically and pharmacologically related to amphetamine

minimal brain syndrome   a relatively mild impairment of brain function that affects perception and behavior

neuron   a cell that conducts electrochemical signals

neurotransmitter   a chemical that travels from the axon of one neuron, across the synaptic gap, and to the receptor site on the dendrite of an adjacent neuron, thus allowing communication between neural cells

norepinephrine   a neurotransmitter in both the central and peripheral nervous systems

opiates   compounds from the milky juice of the poppy plant *Papaver somniferum*, including opium, morphine, codeine, and their derivatives, such as heroin

paranoia   a mental condition characterized by extreme suspiciousness, fear, delusions, and, in extreme cases, hallucinations

parasympathetic nervous system   a subdivision of the autonomic nervous system whose nerves constrict pupils, slow heart rate, and enhance digestive and sexual functioning

peripheral nervous system   neural material outside the brain and spinal cord, including motor and sensory neurons

pharmacology   the study of drugs and their sources, appearance, chemistry, actions, and uses

physical dependence   an adaptation of the body to the presence of a drug such that its absence produces withdrawal symptoms

positive reinforcer   any event or stimulus that results in an increased probability that the behavior that produced it will reoccur in the future

psychological dependence a condition in which the drug user craves a drug to maintain a sense of well-being and feels discomfort when deprived of it

psychomotor stimulant any substance, such as amphetamine, that when ingested produces a general increase in behavioral activity

psychosis a behavioral disorder characterized by a loss of contact with commonly perceived reality and symptoms such as delusions, hallucinations, and emotional and cognitive breakdown

receptor site a specialized area located on a dendrite which, when bound by a sufficient number of neurotransmitter molecules, produces an electrical charge

schizophrenia a chronic psychotic disorder with symptoms such as paranoia, delusions, and hallucinations

sensitization a state of progressively increasing responsiveness to a drug, such that less drug is required to obtain a given response

stress the nonspecific response of the body to any intellectual, emotional, and/or physical demand

sympathetic nervous system the subdivision of the autonomic nervous system stimulated during stress and whose nerves, by releasing epinephrine and norepinephrine, dilate the pupils, accelerate the heart, and inhibit digestive and sexual functioning

synapse the microscopic gap between the axon and dendrite of two adjacent neurons in which neurotransmitters travel

tolerance a decrease of susceptibility to the effects of a drug due to its continued administration, resulting in the user's need to increase the drug dosage in order to achieve the effects experienced previously

tricyclic antidepressants a class of drugs used therapeutically to relieve depression and elevate mood in individuals who are psychologically depressed

vasoconstrictor a substance that acts to constrict or narrow blood vessels

withdrawal the physiological and psychological effects of discontinued usage of a drug

Index

acquired immune deficiency syndrome
(AIDS), 39
see also cocaine, infections and
Adrenalin *see* epinephrine
AIDS *see* acquired immune deficiency
syndrome
alcohol, 39, 55, 60, 63, 81
alkaloids, 20, 65
amphetamines, 23, 33–37, 40–42, 48,
58–59, 63, 73, 78–79, 90, 92
see also cocaine, adulterants and;
cocaine, central nervous system
cocaine, tolerance
amygdala, 35
see also cocaine, central nervous
system
anesthetics, local, 30–32, 40
see also cocaine, anesthetic effect;
cocaine, medical uses
appetite *see* cocaine, anorectic effects
Aschenbrandt, Theodor, 53–54
assertiveness training, 87
see also cocaine, abuse, treatment
autonomic nervous system, 29
see also central nervous system
axon, 31, 78
see also nerves,
barbiturates, 39, 73
base *see* cocaine, base form
Belushi, John, 39
see also cocaine, interactions with
other drugs
Benzedrine, 36
see also amphetamines
biofeedback, 87
see also cocaine, abuse, treatment
"body packing," 38
see also cocaine, smuggling
brain *see* central nervous system
brain stimulation, 77
see also cocaine, animal models for
studying; cocaine, reinforcing
qualities
catecholamines, 78, 89
central nervous system, 29
see also cocaine, central nervous
system; cocaine, psychological
effects; nerves, transmission of
impulses

coca paste, 26, 65, 70, 93
see also cocaine, processing
cocaine
absorption, 22–23, 26
abuse, 19, 45–48, 56–57
treatment, 81–93
abuse potential, 48, 76–77
adulterants and, 23, 26, 40
anesthetic effect, 30, 32, 48
animal models for studying, 73–79
anorectic effects, 34, 40–41
base form, 20–21, 45
cardiovascular system, effects on,
32–33, 37–38, 42
central nervous system, effects on,
22, 24–27, 33–42, 77–79
controlling trafficking, 67, 69, 70–71
dependence, 37, 43–44
dosage, 25–27, 37
economics, 21, 26, 61, 66–67
history, 19, 22–23, 30, 51–59
hotline number for users, 44, 47
hydrochloride salt, 20–21, 24, 26, 65
infections and, 39
interactions with other drugs, 26,
39–40
intranasal administration, 24–25, 59,
62, 82
intravenous administration, 25, 27,
35, 39, 41–42, 62, 82
legal status, 48–49, 57
medical uses, 30, 32, 48, 54–55
metabolism, 37
misconceptions, 19, 44, 55–59
neurotransmitters and, 33–34
oral use, 22–23, 51
paste form, 45, 65
patterns of use
in South America, 22, 26, 93
in United States, 21–22, 37, 57,
59–63
perceptions, 21–22
powder form, 23–24
processing, 20–21, 23, 26, 65–66
psychological effects, 22, 24–27,
35–36, 39, 45–48
psychosis caused by, 36, 39, 57, 79,
83
reasons for using, 62, 82–83

reinforcing qualities, 75–79
routes of administration, 20, 22–27
smoking, 20–21, 26–27, 35–36, 62
smuggling, 23, 38–39, 48–49, 67–71
social problems caused by, 39,
    45–48, 82, 93
tolerance, 40–43
toxic effects, 26–27, 32–39, 44–45,
    57, 76–77
see also Erythroxylon coca;
    freebasing
Coca-Cola, 56
coffee, 52
Conquistadors, 51–52
contingency contracting, 85–86
    see also cocaine, abuse, treatment
Controlled Substances Act, 48
Cousteau, Jacques, 19
"crash," 36
DA *see* dopamine
DEA *see* Drug Enforcement Agency
dependence, physical, 37, 43
    animal models for studying, 73–74
    see also cocaine, dependence
desensitization, 86–87
    see also cocaine, abuse, treatment
Dexedrine, 36
    see also amphetamines
diazepam *see* Valium
diethylpropion, 76
    see also cocaine, reinforcing qualities
dopamine (DA), 33–34, 78–79
    see also neurotransmitters
Drug Abuse Warning Network (DAWN),
    60
Drug Enforcement Agency (DEA), 39, 48,
    70
    see also cocaine, controlling
        trafficking
drug schedules, 48, 58
    see also cocaine, legal status
Edison, Thomas, 56
EEG *see* electroencephalograph
electroencephalograph (EEG), 35, 41
    see also cocaine, central nervous
        system
epilepsy, 35, 38–39, 79
    see also cocaine, central nervous
        system
epinephrine, 33

see also neurotransmitters
erythroxyline, 53
Erythroxylon coca, 20, 65
euphoria, 24, 26, 35–36, 43, 77, 79,
    90–91
    see also cocaine, psychological
        effects
FDA *see* Food and Drug Administration
Fleischl-Marxow, Ernst von, 56–57
Food and Drug Administration (FDA), 48,
    58
    see also cocaine, legal status
freebasing, 20–21, 26–27, 62, 82
    see also cocaine, processing; cocaine,
        smoking; cocaine, toxic effects
Freud, Sigmund, 19, 30, 54–57
    see also cocaine, history
Gaedecke (German chemist), 53
ginseng, 89
    see also cocaine, abuse, treatment
glucose, 89
    see also cocaine, abuse, treatment
hallucinations, 26, 36, 84
    see also cocaine, central nervous
        system; cocaine, psychological
        effects; cocaine, psychosis
        caused by; cocaine, toxic effects
Harrison Narcotic Act, 48, 57
hepatitis B, 39
heroin, 39, 43, 60, 73, 92
    see also cocaine, interactions with
        other drugs; speedballing
hydrotherapy, 87
    see also cocaine, abuse, treatment
hyperactivity, 91
    see also methylphenidate
hyperthermia, 38, 40
    see also cocaine, central nervous
        system
Incas, 51–52
Indians, Peruvian, 19, 22
kindling, 35
    see also cocaine, central nervous
        system
Koller, Carl, 30
limbic system, 35, 79
    see also cocaine, central nervous
        system
lithium, 90–91
    see also cocaine, abuse, treatment

marijuana, 26, 39, 60, 62–63
MBD *see* minimal brain dysfunction
methadone, 92
methaqualone, 39
methylphenidate, 91–92
    see also cocaine, abuse, treatment
minimal brain dysfunction, 91–92
    see also cocaine, abuse, treatment
morphine, 55–56, 81
National Commission on Marijuana and
        Drug Abuse, 58–59
National Household Survey, 60
    see also cocaine, patterns of use in
        United States
National Institute of Drug Abuse, 60
    see also cocaine, patterns of use in
        United States
NE *see* norepinephrine
nerves, 30–32
    see also central nervous system;
        cocaine, anesthetic effect
neuron *see* nerves
neurotransmitters, 31–33, 78–79
    see also cocaine, central nervous
        system; nerves
Niemann, Albert, 53
norepinephrine (NE), 33–34, 78–79
Novocaine, 30
    see also anesthetics, local
nucleus accumbens, 79
    see also cocaine, reinforcing qualities
1-tryptophan, 89
    see also cocaine, abuse, treatment
opiates, 63
    see also heroin; morphine
opium, 55, 57
parasympathetic nervous system, 29
peripheral nervous system, 29
phenylpropanolamine, 89
    see also cocaine, abuse, treatment
positive reinforcers, 74
    see also cocaine, animal models for
        studying; cocaine, reinforcing
        qualities
procaine, 76
    see also anesthetics, local; cocaine,
        reinforcing qualities
Pryor, Richard, 27
pseudocholinesterases, 37
    see also cocaine, toxic effects

Quaaludes *see* methaqualone
receptors, 31, 33, 78–79, 90
    see also neurotransmitters
Ritalin *see* methylphenidate
"rush," 25, 27, 35–36
    see also cocaine, psychological
        effects
schizophrenia, 36, 79
    see also cocaine, psychosis caused by
self-help techniques, 88–89
    see also cocaine, abuse, treatment
septicemia, 39
Smith, D. E., 59
"snorting," 24
    see also cocaine, intranasal
        administration
"speedballing," 39, 60
    see also cocaine, interactions with
        other drugs
spinal cord *see* central nervous system
stereotypy, 33–34, 42
    see also cocaine, central nervous
        system
subacute bacterial endocarditis, 39
sympathetic nervous system, 29, 33
synapses, 31, 78
    see also nerves
synergism, 39
tea, 52
Thorazine, 84
    see also cocaine, abuse, treatment
tobacco, 26, 52
    see also cocaine, interactions with
        other drugs
tolerance *see* cocaine, tolerance
tranquilizers, 39, 60, 63
tricyclic antidepressants, 90
    see also cocaine, abuse, treatment
tyrosine, 89
    see also cocaine, abuse, treatment
Uber Coca (Freud), 54
Valium, 84
    see also cocaine, abuse, treatment
Verne, Jules, 56
Vin Mariani, 56
vitamin C, 89
    see also cocaine, abuse, treatment
Wesson, D. R., 59
Wöhler, Friedrich, 53

Chris-Ellyn Johanson, Ph.D., received her degree in psychology from the University of Chicago. Dr. Johanson is an associate professor of psychiatry at the University of Chicago Medical School and is associate director of the Drug Abuse Research Center. She is a former president of the International Study Group Investigating Drugs as Reinforcers.

Solomon H. Snyder, M.D., is Distinguished Service Professor of Neuroscience, Pharmacology and Psychiatry at The Johns Hopkins University School of Medicine. He has served as president of the Society for Neuroscience and in 1978 received the Albert Lasker Award in Medical Research. He has authored *Uses of Marijuana, Madness and the Brain, The Troubled Mind, Biological Aspects of Mental Disorder,* and edited *Perspective in Neuropharmacology: A Tribute to Julius Axelrod.* Professor Snyder was a research associate with Dr. Axelrod at the National Institute of Health.

Barry L. Jacobs, Ph.D., is currently a professor in the program of neuroscience at Princeton University. Professor Jacobs is author of *Serotinin Neurotransmission and Behavior* and *Hallucinogens: Neurochemical, Behavioral and Clinical Perspectives.* He has written many journal articles in the field of neuroscience and contributed numerous chapters to books on behavior and brain science. He has been a member of several panels of the National Institute of Mental Health.

Jerome H. Jaffe, M.D., formerly professor of psychiatry at the College of Physicians and Surgeons, Columbia University, has been named recently Director of the Addiction Research Center of the National Institute on Drug Abuse. Dr. Jaffe is also a psychopharmacologist and has conducted research on a wide range of addictive drugs and developed treatment programs for addicts. He has acted as Special Consultant to the President on Narcotics and Dangerous Drugs and was the first director of the White House Special Action Office for Drug Abuse Prevention.